Health Issues for Young People

ISSUES

Volume 176

Series Editor

Lisa Firth

Independence

Educational Publishers
Cambridge

First published by Independence
The Studio, High Green
Great Shelford
Cambridge CB22 5EG
England

© Independence 2009

British Library Cataloguing in Publication Data
Health Issues for Young People – (Issues; v.176)
1. Teenagers – Health and hygiene 2. Health behavior in adolescence
I. Series II. Firth, Lisa
613'.0433-dc22

ISBN-13: 978 1 86168 500 1

Printed in Great Britain
MWL Print Group Ltd

Cover
The illustration on the front cover is by
Don Hatcher.

CONTENTS

Chapter One: Healthy Lifestyles

Chapter Two: Sexual Health

Chapter Three: Mental Health

Useful information for readers

Dear Reader,

Issues: Health Issues for Young People

At a time when three in ten children in Britain are overweight or obese and the UK has the third highest number of 15 and 16 year olds with an alcohol problem, how do young people deal with the health issues associated with their age group? This books looks at nutrition and exercise, mental health problems including depression, eating disorders and self-harm, and the prevalence of risk-taking behaviours such as smoking, binge drinking, drug use and unsafe sex.

The purpose of *Issues*

Health Issues for Young People is the one hundred and seventy-sixth volume in the **Issues** series. The aim of this series is to offer up-to-date information about important issues in our world. Whether you are a regular reader or new to the series, we do hope you find this book a useful overview of the many and complex issues involved in the topic. This title replaces an older volume in the **Issues** series, Volume 123: **Young People and Health**, which is now out of print.

Titles in the **Issues** series are resource books designed to be of especial use to those undertaking project work or requiring an overview of facts, opinions and information on a particular subject, particularly as a prelude to undertaking their own research.

The information in this book is not from a single author, publication or organisation; the value of this unique series lies in the fact that it presents information from a wide variety of sources, including:

⇨ Government reports and statistics
⇨ Newspaper articles and features
⇨ Information from think-tanks and policy institutes
⇨ Magazine features and surveys
⇨ Website material
⇨ Literature from lobby groups and charitable organisations.*

Critical evaluation

Because the information reprinted here is from a number of different sources, readers should bear in mind the origin of the text and whether the source is likely to have a particular bias or agenda when presenting information (just as they would if undertaking their own research). It is hoped that, as you read about the many aspects of the issues explored in this book, you will critically evaluate the information presented. It is important that you decide whether you are being presented with facts or opinions. Does the writer give a biased or an unbiased report? If an opinion is being expressed, do you agree with the writer?

Health Issues for Young People offers a useful starting point for those who need convenient access to information about the many issues involved. However, it is only a starting point. Following each article is a URL to the relevant organisation's website, which you may wish to visit for further information.

Kind regards,

Lisa Firth
Editor, **Issues** series

** Please note that Independence Publishers has no political affiliations or opinions on the topics covered in the **Issues** series, and any views quoted in this book are not necessarily those of the publisher or its staff.*

ISSUES TODAY
A RESOURCE FOR KEY STAGE 3

Younger readers can also benefit from the thorough editorial process which characterises the **Issues** series with our resource books for 11- to 14-year-old students, **Issues Today**. In addition to containing information from a wide range of sources, rewritten with this age group in mind, **Issues Today** titles also feature comprehensive glossaries, an accessible and attractive layout and handy tasks and assignments which can be used in class, for homework or as a revision aid. In addition, these titles are fully photocopiable. For more information, please visit our website (www.independence. co.uk).

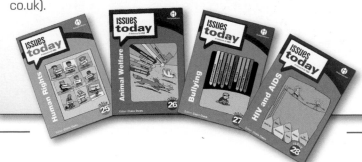

Health questionnaire

How healthy is your lifestyle?

Please answer this questionnaire by responding 'always', 'usually', 'sometimes' or 'never' for each question.

Then, add up your points and 'score' your questionnaire.

Finally, answer the 'What do you think and know about your health?' questions.

Questions

1 Do you eat a balanced diet, low in sugar and fat?
2 Do you eat five portions of vegetables each day?
3 Do you eat some fruit each day?
4 Are you happy with your body size and shape?
5 Do you drink about six glasses of water a day?
6 Do you avoid drinking sugary drinks?
7 Do you get enough sleep (about 8-10 hours a night)?
8 Do you brush your teeth daily?
9 Do you go to the dentist regularly for a check up?
10 Do you have a sensible balance between rest, school and play?
11 Are you a non-smoker?
12 Are you calm and controlled?
13 Do you have a few good friends?
14 Do you do about 60 minutes of activity each day?
15 Do you think you are a healthy person?
16 Do you think you are an active person?
17 Do you think you are fit?
18 Would you describe yourself as happy?

Calculating your healthy lifestyle score

You score:
⇨ 4 points for each 'always' response.
⇨ 3 points for each 'usually' response.
⇨ 2 points for each 'sometimes' response.
⇨ 1 point for each 'never' response.

Over 60
Congratulations, you lead a very healthy lifestyle and will benefit from this now and in the future. Keep up the good work and try and influence your friends to be as healthy as you!

Between 40 and 59
Well done, you are healthy much of the time and will be benefiting from this. You might consider becoming even healthier by changing some of your lifestyle habits.

Between 21 and 39
This is okay but could be much better. You are healthy some of the time and will be benefiting from this. However, you might consider becoming healthier by improving on a number of your lifestyle habits.

Less than 20
Oh dear, you lead an unhealthy lifestyle and are likely to suffer because of this now and in later in life. You might consider becoming much healthier by improving many of your lifestyle habits.

What do you think and know about your health?

What you know about your health
What does your healthy lifestyle score tell you?
⇨ What have you done well on?
⇨ What have you not done as well on?

What you think about your health
⇨ Do you think you need to become healthier? If yes, in what ways?
⇨ What do you think you can change about your lifestyle?

Health plans
State three things (actions) you could do over the next three months to improve your health and lifestyle.
⇨ What will help you to do these things (actions)?
⇨ What might stop you from doing these things (actions)?

On a scale of 0-10, how confident are you that you will be able to improve your fitness levels over the next three months?

⇨ The above information is reprinted with kind permission from Healthy Schools. Visit www.healthyschools.gov.uk for more information on this and other related topics.

© Crown copyright

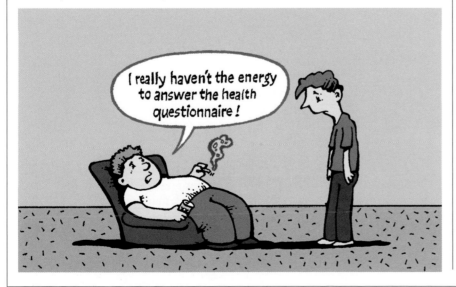

I really haven't the energy to answer the health questionnaire!

How healthy are our children?

New evidence from the latest Health Survey for England

Most children in England are not obese or overweight, meet the government's recommended physical activity targets, don't smoke or drink and think healthy food is enjoyable – although they're not reaching the 'five a day' target – according to the latest Health Survey for England (HSE).

The annual survey, conducted in 2007 by researchers at UCL (University College London) and the National Centre for Social Research (NatCen) and funded by The NHS Information Centre, has its latest results published today. It draws on data from interviews and measurements of thousands of people representative of the whole population.

The HSE 2007 had a particular focus on children, including data from over 7,500 2-15 year olds. Those old enough were interviewed about their knowledge and attitudes concerning key aspects of lifestyle including smoking, drinking, eating and physical activity.

The survey also collected data about the impact of smokefree legislation brought in on 1 July 2007. This indicates that although the number of adults and children smoking had not decreased at this early stage, there were some positive initial signs of a reduction in cigarette consumption and in children's exposure to smoke.

Dr Nicola Shelton, Senior Lecturer in UCL's Department of Epidemiology and Public Health and an editor of the study, said:

'Behaviours and attitudes towards personal health formed early in life extend into later childhood and adulthood, ultimately having an impact on health over an individual's lifespan. It's crucial we understand children's attitudes and behaviour about issues such as exercise, diet and smoking because their early experiences have such an influence going into adulthood.

'Although the survey shows a mixed picture for both children and adults, and we're still seeing marked differences in the health of different socio-economic groups, there's quite a lot to be positive about here – for instance, the initial signs that the rising childhood and adult obesity trend could be beginning to level out – although we're not seeing the decline we'd hoped for.

'Another potential positive result is that children's cotinine levels (indicating exposure to tobacco smoke) did not increase after 1 July, when smokefree legislation was introduced. Some people had been worried that the legislation would cause adults to smoke more at home and children would experience greater exposure – our results do not reflect this.

'Despite the positives, there's no room for complacency and the momentum to keep improving the nation's health must continue.'

Rachel Craig, Research Director for the Health Survey for England at NatCen, and co-editor of the report, added:

'In the 2007 Health Survey we can compare behaviour with knowledge and attitudes, and there are some interesting differences. Like adults, more children know about fruit and vegetable targets than meet them. More children think they are very or fairly active than do the recommended amount of physical activity.

'We need to continue making people aware of the targets they should aim for to achieve a healthier lifestyle. Parents are an important influence on their children, so we should make sure the right messages get through to them as well as to children and young people.' The key findings about children from the HSE 2007 include:

Obesity

⇨ According to BMI measurements, around three in ten boys and girls aged 2-15 were either overweight or obese.

⇨ There are indications that the continuing rise in levels of obesity amongst children may have begun to flatten out.

⇨ Children aged 11-15 classed as obese were more likely to say they want to do more physical activity than those of normal weight.

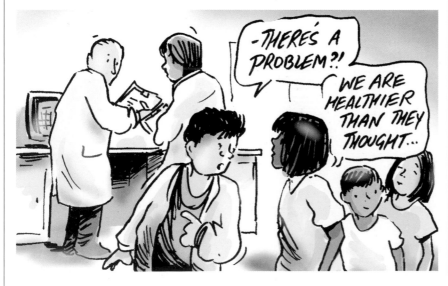

Physical activity

⇨ More boys than girls met government physical activity targets (72 per cent and 63 per cent, respectively).

⇨ For girls, the proportion meeting the target steadily declined after the age of nine.

⇨ Most boys and girls aged 11-15 perceived themselves to be either very or fairly physically active compared with other people their age (90 per cent and 84 per cent respectively). This includes 68 per cent of boys and 67 per cent of girls in the least active group, who thought they were very or fairly physically active compared with others.

⇨ Girls aged 11-15 were more likely than boys of the same age to want to do more physical activity (74 per cent and 61 per cent respectively). This proportion declined with age among boys, but not among girls.

Diet and healthy eating

⇨ Among children aged 5-15, 21 per cent of both boys and girls reached the 'five a day' target for fruit and vegetables – a similar proportion to adults.

⇨ 63 per cent of boys and 73 per cent of girls aged 11-15 knew that five portions of fruit and vegetables should be eaten each day. However, only 22 per cent of boys and 21 per cent of girls could correctly identify what a portion was.

⇨ Most children aged 11-15 thought their diet was 'quite healthy' (70 per cent of boys and 72 per cent of girls), and only one per cent of children thought their diet was 'very unhealthy'.

⇨ The majority of children aged 11-15 agreed that 'Healthy foods are enjoyable', with more girls than boys agreeing with the statement (72 per cent compared with 64 per cent).

Smoking

⇨ Only two per cent of children aged 8-15 reported they were regular smokers (at least one cigarette a week). This was higher among older children, with eight per cent of boys and ten per cent of girls aged 15 reporting that they smoked regularly.

⇨ 20 per cent of those aged 15 had a cotinine level of 15ng/ml or more (indicative of smoking), but only nine per cent reported that they were regular smokers.

⇨ No differences were found in self-reported smoking behaviour or cotinine levels before and after the introduction of the smokefree legislation in England on 1 July 2007 – this applied to both children and adults. The proportion of children aged 0-12 who were exposed to smoke by a carer for two or more hours a week was lower than in 2006.

Alcohol

⇨ 35 per cent of boys and 34 per cent of girls aged 8-15 reported having experience of drinking alcohol.

⇨ Frequency of drinking was clearly related to age, increasing from seven per cent of boys and eight per cent of girls aged eight to 79 per cent of boys and 74 per cent of girls aged 15.

⇨ Girls aged 13-15 were slightly more likely than boys of this age to agree that: 'People of my age drink to be sociable with friends' (73 per cent and 66 per cent respectively). More than half of both boys and girls aged 13-15 agreed that young people drink because of pressure from friends (56 per cent of girls and 53 per cent of boys).

16 December 2008

⇨ The above information is reprinted with kind permission from the National Centre for Social Research. Visit www.natcen.ac.uk for more.

© *NatCen*

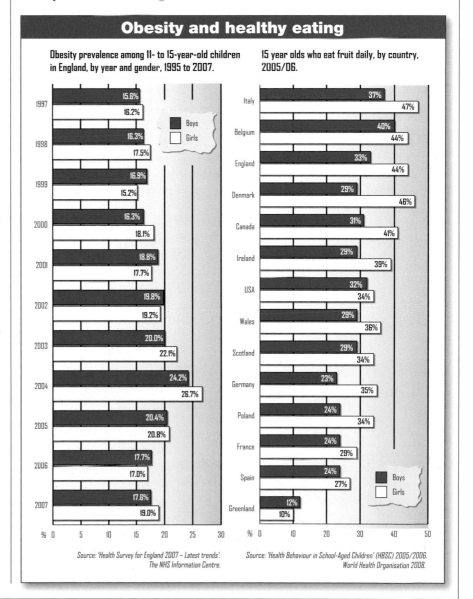

Obesity and healthy eating

Obesity prevalence among 11- to 15-year-old children in England, by year and gender, 1995 to 2007.

Year	Boys	Girls
1997	15.6%	16.2%
1998	16.3%	17.5%
1999	16.9%	15.2%
2000	16.3%	18.1%
2001	18.8%	17.7%
2002	19.8%	19.2%
2003	20.0%	22.1%
2004	24.2%	26.7%
2005	20.4%	20.8%
2006	17.7%	17.0%
2007	17.6%	19.0%

Source: 'Health Survey for England 2007 – Latest trends'. The NHS Information Centre.

15 year olds who eat fruit daily, by country, 2005/06.

Country	Boys	Girls
Italy	37%	47%
Belgium	40%	44%
England	33%	44%
Denmark	29%	46%
Canada	31%	41%
Ireland	29%	39%
USA	32%	34%
Wales	29%	36%
Scotland	29%	34%
Germany	23%	35%
Poland	24%	34%
France	24%	29%
Spain	24%	27%
Greenland	12%	10%

Source: 'Health Behaviour in School-Aged Children' (HBSC) 2005/2006. World Health Organisation 2008.

Adolescent health

10 facts on adolescent health

The state of adolescent health

One in every five people in the world is an adolescent, and 85% of them live in developing countries. Nearly two-thirds of premature deaths and one-third of the total disease burden in adults are associated with conditions or behaviours that began in youth, including tobacco use, a lack of physical activity, unprotected sex or exposure to violence. Promoting healthy practices during adolescence, and efforts that better protect this age group from risks will ensure longer, more productive lives for many.

HIV and young people

Young people aged 15-24 accounted for an estimated 45% of new HIV infections worldwide in 2007. They need to know how to protect themselves from HIV and have the means to do so. Better access to testing and counselling will inform young people about their HIV status, help them get the care they need, and avoid further spread of the virus.

Early pregnancy and childbirth

About 16 million girls aged 15-19 give birth every year – roughly 11% of all births worldwide. The vast majority of births to adolescents occur in developing countries. The risk of dying from pregnancy-related causes is much higher for adolescents than for older women. Laws and community actions that support a minimum age for marriage, as well as better access to contraception, can decrease too-early pregnancies.

Malnutrition

Many boys and girls in developing countries enter adolescence undernourished, making them more vulnerable to disease and early death. Conversely, overweight and obesity – another form of malnutrition with serious health consequences – is increasing among other young people in both low- and high-income countries. Adequate nutrition and healthy eating and physical exercise habits at this age are foundations for good health in adulthood.

Mental health

At least 20% of young people will experience some form of mental illness – such as depression, mood disturbances, substance abuse, suicidal behaviours or eating disorders. Promoting mental health, and responding to problems if they arise requires a range of adolescent-friendly health care and counselling services in communities.

20% of young people will experience some form of mental illness

---

Tobacco use

The vast majority of tobacco users worldwide begin during adolescence. Today more than 150 million adolescents use tobacco, and this number is increasing globally. Bans on tobacco advertising, raising the prices of tobacco products, and laws that prohibit smoking in public places reduce the number of people who start using tobacco products. They furthermore lower the amount of tobacco consumed by smokers and increase the numbers of young people who quit smoking.

Harmful drinking of alcohol

Harmful drinking among young people is an increasing concern in many countries. It reduces self-control and increases risky behaviours. Harmful drinking is a primary cause of injuries (including those due to road traffic accidents), violence (especially domestic violence), and premature deaths. Regulating access to alcohol is an effective strategy to reduce harmful use by young people. Bans on alcohol advertising can lessen peer pressure on adolescents to drink.

Violence

Among 15-19 year olds, suicide is the second leading cause of death, followed by violence in the community and family. Promoting nurturing relations between parents and children early in life, training in life skills, and reducing access to alcohol and lethal means such as firearms can help prevent violence. More effective and sensitive care for adolescent victims of violence is needed.

Injuries and road safety

Unintentional injuries are a leading cause of death and disability in adolescents; and road traffic injuries, drowning and burns are the most common types. Injury rates among adolescents are highest in developing countries, and within countries, they are more likely to occur among adolescents from poorer families. Community actions to promote road safety (including the passing of safety laws that are well enforced) and public education targeted to young people on how to avoid drowning, burns and falls can reduce injuries.

WHO response

Many adolescent health challenges are closely interrelated and successful interventions in one area can lead to positive outcomes in other areas. WHO is helping countries:
⇨ to collect, analyse and use data on adolescent health to support and inform policy-making;
⇨ to develop evidence-based policies and programmes that support adolescent health;
⇨ to increase access to and use of health services for adolescents;
⇨ to strengthen contributions from the education, media and other sectors to improve adolescent health.

September 2008

⇨ The above information is reprinted with kind permission from the World Health Organisation. Visit www.who.int for more information.

© WHO

'Is drinking too much really that big a deal?'

Should you have a sexual health check? Must you find a new GP? And will people know if you're a virgin? Dr Adam Connor, a university doctor, answers some frequently asked questions

When I'm feeling ill, I tell my mum and she looks after me or calls the doctor. Who should I tell at university if I'm not well?

There may be specific GP practices where you can register, or even a practice on the campus. If you are ill, make an appointment with the GP or ring your practice to ask for advice. If you feel ill and your practice is closed, then there will be an emergency GP service, or alternatively ring NHS Direct for advice on 0845 4647.

When you are unwell, make sure someone locally knows, so they can look in on you and make sure you're not getting a lot worse.

My boyfriend and I have been going out since year 11, but we've decided to break up when we go to uni. Should I have a sexual health check-up?

It is a good time to do this, and essential if you have any symptoms. If you have any concerns, have a sexual-health screen. Some student-based practices have developed their own services. Always use condoms with new or casual partners and continue with this until you are sure you and your established partner have no STIs.

Is drinking too much really that big a deal? University is only for three years.

Getting drunk now and then is not harmful, but there are degrees of danger. In the short term, the risks are not from the physical effects of alcohol but from related accidents.

Emergency departments are full of people who have hurt themselves or been hurt by others when drunk. Unfortunately, I have seen countless students (male and female) who describe truly horrible circumstances of assault (physical and sexual) that have occurred only because they were so drunk. Drink (if you wish), be happy and enjoy, but make sure you stay safe.

I honestly think I might be exam-phobic. I find the whole experience of doing an exam absolutely crippling. Am I stupid to be even going to university?

Most students feel stressed at some time about something. Exam fears are normal. It's true that some feel it more than others, and some even get to the point of feeling ill, but this mustn't stop you going to university. If you really struggle with exams, there are tactics you can use to build up to them. The university will have a student support section that will help students who feel like this. In extreme cases, anxiety can have physical symptoms (feeling your heart race, difficulty sleeping, etc). Consult your GP if this is the case.

It is so hard to get on a doctor's list at home. I don't want to register with a GP at university; do I have to?

There can be a number of reasons why students don't want to move practice. However, the NHS asks that you are registered with a GP near your term address. Statistically, you are much more likely to get ill in term time than when on holiday. Your notes and past history are really helpful to a GP, and it can take six to eight weeks for notes to transfer, so register with a GP as soon as possible. Obviously, if you have longer-term conditions it is even more important.

I'm really scared of going to university, as I find it very hard to make new friends. Will I fit in?

Most people feel out of place when starting university – it can feel a very big step. Just about everybody agrees that this is one of the best bits about university life, developing your own independence and your own identity in a way you've not been able to before.

Not everyone has the confidence to start speaking to people they've not met before, but give yourself the best chance by participating in clubs that interest you.

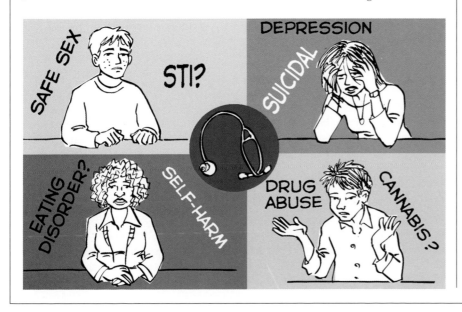

I never do serious drugs, but me and my mates share the occasional spliff and I've done a few pills. I'd never touch any hard drugs. That's OK, isn't it?

Because you've got away with it so far does not mean it is without risk. There is increasing evidence of a long-term effect on mental health for people who use cannabis. And with 'pills' you don't know what you're getting. These are illegal substances and therefore they are beyond any controls. You don't get a list of what's in it or a use-by date.

Both these types of drugs can form into a habit easily. They have physical dependence properties, but the main difficulty is with social habit – 'this is what I do when I go out'. The social habit can lead to problems in your life. University is a clean break from home so now may be a good time to choose not to use these substances.

I've had depression since I was 14 and the doctor put me on tablets last year. I'm worried how this will affect my time at university.

If your doctor thought you should be on these tablets, then you should remain on them for now. Make an appointment to see your new doctor at university. It may be worth booking a longer appointment so you go through the past history. Don't just stop them on your own. Take advice and ensure someone is continuing to see that your mood is ok. Usually anti-depressants help with low mood, which can cause loss of concentration, poor memory and lack of sleep. So, being on the tablets may make you work and function better than if you came off them.

I think I may have an eating disorder. I'm worried people will notice at university.

Many eating disorders are linked with a common theme of control. Some of the students I see have had issues for years, but eventually resolve the problems themselves. However, there is help available no matter how serious the problem is or how long it's been going on. Speak to your GP, or a counsellor, or explore local services for eating disorders – NHS Direct can help with this.

Everyone else seems to have done everything. They smoke and drink and have had loads of girls. I am so straight; I really don't think I'll fit in. What if a girl realises I'm a virgin?

You are not a lesser person than someone else because your experiences have been different. Just be you. You've no need to lie, but equally no need to share or broadcast your experiences or lack of them.

No girl or boy can tell what you have or haven't done and they are not likely to ask you (many of them will feel like you do and worry what you might say in return). Your best defence in any potential relationship is to pick someone you really get on with on lots of different levels. As for your mates, say nothing – most guys will tease each other about different things, and sex is a common target. But ride it out – there'll be others hearing the same jokes and jibes, hoping no one asks them.

⇨ Dr Adam Connor is a GP at the University of Nottingham health service.

14 August 2008

What's the best exercise for teenagers?

Information from NHS Choices

Exercise isn't always at the top of your daily agenda if you're a teenager. Today's world is saturated with activities that mean keeping fit can feel like a drag.

Social networking, watching TV, or downloading the latest tunes onto your MP3 player can leave little room for exercising. However, there are several health and lifestyle benefits to maintaining a regular exercise routine, such as lowering your risk of heart disease and giving you more energy.

Keeping yourself fit

You should try to do at least 60 minutes of moderate-intensity exercise a day. If this sounds a little overwhelming then break this time up into three lots of 20-minute activities, for example:

⇨ start with a 20-minute brisk walk to the shops;

⇨ ride your bike to the park instead of catching the bus; and

⇨ finish the day with a game of frisbee in the garden.

Activities can be broken up into two categories, aerobic exercise and strength training. Both are important to any exercise routine, but try to alternate between them:

⇨ Aerobic exercises – such as jogging, swimming and playing tennis. This kind of exercise can be strenuous (demanding) on your body, so try not to overdo it. Remember to always warm up before, and warm down after any form of exercise.

⇨ Strength training (also know as resistance training) – such as lifting weights and using machines to improve your muscle strength. Always start this type of exercise under the supervision of a trained professional, such as a coach or fitness trainer at a gym. This way you'll learn how to do the exercises properly and avoid hurting yourself.

Get active

A five-year study carried out by Cancer Research UK found that physical activity declined in both teenage girls and boys, while sedentary (deskbound) activities increased. This imbalance can lead you to gain weight, meaning it is likely you will have health problems in later life, such as type two diabetes (your body doesn't make enough insulin).

The study, also supported by the British Heart Foundation, found that the average viewing time of 16 year olds was 16 hours a week. If you feel you're spending too much time in front of the TV or computer, it's never too late to get active and take control of your health and weight.

If you want to get fit, why not consider joining a gym? Most gyms in the UK allow people as young as 13 to become members. However, at this age you will not be able to use the weights, and it's likely you'll be supervised during your first few sessions. Exercising at a gym isn't for everyone. You may instead prefer to join a local sports centre to swim, or take part in aerobic classes.

If you feel like being sociable why not try some group sports? Most can be played down the local park, or ask at your local sports centre about team activities you can take part in. You could try your hand at squash, hockey, badminton, or even martial arts. If this sounds a little intensive, why not try dance classes or table tennis. Group sports can also help you develop important team-building skills.

Keeping fit doesn't always have to be about taking up sports or joining classes. Getting active round the house will not only improve your health, but also help you gain brownie points with the folks! Why not help to vacuum the house, clean out the garage, cut the lawn, or even tidy your room to build up a sweat!

Control your weight

Keeping your waistline under control involves making sure you eat a healthy balanced diet, as well as doing regular exercise. It's important to remember that exercise not only burns fat, but also:

⇨ helps tone and firm up your body,

⇨ makes you feel more energised, and
⇨ ensures you maintain a healthy metabolism – minimising your need to restrict your diet.

In the UK it's believed one out of four 11-15 year olds are overweight. Being overweight at a young age increases your risk of developing serious health problems, such as coronary artery disease (having blocked arteries) and high blood pressure (narrow arteries). If these health problems are not addressed immediately it is likely you will have them throughout your adult life.

Boost your image

Not only can exercise help reduce your risk to all kinds of heart-related illness in later life, it can also help clear up your spots! Exercise naturally boosts the circulation in your skin, which helps to keep spots and acne at bay.

Exercise can also help you combat those unwanted lumps and bumps by firming up your muscles. Feeling confident in your own skin can help you maintain an active lifestyle.

On a more serious note, being overweight can also have psychological affects on how you feel. You may begin to feel isolated and depressed, or even start to develop a negative body image (how you feel about your physical appearance).

Exercise can help if you have anxieties about your body image, but it's important to remember that your body is still growing and changes will continue to happen. How you feel about your body is a very personal thing, and can also change from day to day. If you have any concerns about your body image, speak to someone you trust, such as a family member, close friend, or even your GP.

⇨ The above information is reprinted with kind permission from NHS Choices. Visit www.nhs.uk for more information.

© Crown copyright

Being obese is as bad as a packet of cigarettes

Information from the British Heart Foundation

A new study has suggested that being overweight or seriously underweight as a teenager curbs life expectancy as much as smoking ten cigarettes a day.

Swedish researchers followed 46,000 men from the age of 18 for 38 years. Being obese or smoking more than ten a day doubled the premature death risk.

Being overweight, seriously underweight or smoking ten or less raised it by 30% – and interestingly the fat non-smoker ran the same risk as the fat smoker.

In response to the research paper published by the BMJ Online, Betty McBride, Policy & Communications Director at the British Heart Foundation, said: 'This shocking research found that obese adolescents were at the same risk of an early death as someone with a ten a day plus habit.

'This is an alarming illustration to young people who may have been blasé about the implications of obesity to their future health. The Government needs to bring the same level of sustained focus to tackling the obesity crisis it has previously brought to smoking.

'The number of young people who are overweight and obese is growing. Without tackling this now we risk the next generation growing up with more health problems than their parents.'
25 February 2009

⇨ The above information is reprinted with kind permission from the British Heart Foundation. Visit bhf.org.uk for more information.

© British Heart Foundation 2009

Good nutrition during the teenage years

Healthy eating during your teenage years is essential for supporting the growing body and at this stage the need for most nutrients increases

Your teenage years are one of the fastest growth periods of your life. Physical changes such as puberty affect your body's nutritional needs, while changes in lifestyle may influence eating habits and food choices. Healthy eating during adolescence is essential for supporting the growing body and for preventing future health problems. At this stage, the need for most nutrients increases – particularly calories, protein, calcium and iron.

Calories

Teenagers require approximately 200 more calories than the average adult to provide energy for their growth and generally higher levels of activity. Boys aged 11 to 18 need between 2,500 and 2,800 calories each day and teenage girls need approximately 2,200 calories each day. To meet these calorie needs, teens should choose a variety of healthy foods as shown in the eatwell plate, with the majority of their calorie requirements coming from starchy carbohydrate foods such as potatoes, wholegrain bread and pasta.

Protein

Protein is essential during your teenage years as your body undergoes growth spurts and muscle is developed. Teens need between 45-60g of protein each day and this requirement can easily be met with a good intake of meat, fish and poultry, eggs, dairy products and vegetarian protein sources such as soy products like tofu, Quorn, nuts and seeds. A cup of milk or 25g of red meat contains about 10g of protein; 60g of chopped walnuts contains approximately 15g of protein and 250g of beans provides 12g of protein.

Calcium and vitamin D

Good calcium intake during the teenage years is crucial for maintaining healthy bones and teeth as 90% of our bones are fully formed before the age of 18.

Good sources of calcium include:
- dairy products such as milk, cheese and yogurt;
- seeds such as sesame and sunflower seeds;
- leafy, green vegetables;
- dried fruit;
- sardines;
- fortified foods such as some brands of breakfast cereals, bread and orange juice.

In order to get the required 800-1000mg of calcium per day, try to eat four servings of calcium-rich foods each day, where one serving could include:

Calcium-rich food	Portion size	Approximate amount of calcium
tinned sardines (with bones) in tomato sauce	2-3 sardines (around 60g)	260mg
milk (skimmed or semi-skimmed)	an average glass (200ml)	240mg
cheese	a matchbox-sized piece (125g)	210mg
yogurt	an individual pot (125g)	185mg
sesame seeds	2 tablespoons (25g)	130mg
dried figs	4 fruit (50g)	125mg

Tips for eating calcium-rich foods:
- when choosing dairy products, go for the lower-fat varieties – these have at least the same amount of calcium as higher-fat products while helping you to avoid excess saturated fat and calories
- try stirring sesame seeds or dried fruit into yogurt or add to cereal to further boost your calcium intake.

Vitamin D is needed for the efficient absorption and use of calcium.

Good sources of vitamin D include:
- oily fish such as herring, mackerel or sardines;
- egg yolks;
- fortified foods such as margarine and some brands of breakfast cereals and milk.

Vitamin D is also made by the skin on exposure to sunlight, so try to get outdoors away from the TV and computer games!

Iron and vitamin C

Muscle mass increases during the teenage years so more iron is needed in the diet to keep that developing muscle provided with oxygen. Teenage boys need approximately 12mg of iron each day while girls at this age have exceptionally high iron requirements (15mg/day) due to the onset of menstruation.

Good sources of iron include:
- meat such as beef, lamb and pork;
- pulses such as beans, peas and lentils;
- dried fruits such as prunes, raisins and apricots;
- leafy green vegetables such as spinach;
- fortified foods such as some brands of breakfast cereals.

Very high fibre foods and tea and coffee can reduce your body's ability to absorb iron so try not to eat these at the same time as having iron-rich foods. Do, however, try to eat foods rich in vitamin C along with your iron-rich foods as iron absorption is boosted by this vitamin.

Good sources of vitamin C include:
- citrus, kiwi fruit and berries;
- tomatoes, peppers and leafy green vegetables such as broccoli, brussels sprouts and spinach.

If possible, when your Mum or Dad (or perhaps you!) are preparing the dinner, steam the vegetables, microwave them or boil for a short time in only a little water, as cooking reduces their vitamin C content.

Healthy habits!

Teenagers experiment with food for many reasons, not just their nutritional content. These can include slimming, peer pressure to consume certain brands, the development of personal choice (becoming vegetarian or eating junk food, for example) or consuming a strict diet and supplements to enhance sporting achievements. It is important, then, to get into healthy habits from a young age – healthy family habits can help support the teenager in the family:

⇨ eat a good breakfast;
⇨ eat a variety of foods;
⇨ aim to eat at least five portions of fruit and veg a day;
⇨ have a good intake of calcium- and iron-rich foods;
⇨ choose a diet with plenty of wholegrain products;
⇨ aim for healthy weight;
⇨ be aware of portion sizes;
⇨ limit high fat foods;
⇨ choose a diet moderate in sugars and salt;
⇨ read food labels;
⇨ stay active.

All over the world, teenage and child obesity is on the rise and this has led to an increase in obesity-related diseases

---

Risk of obesity, diabetes and heart disease in teenagers

If you are young and overweight, you are more likely to be overweight or obese as an adult. All over the world, teenage and child obesity is on the rise and this has led to an increase in obesity-related diseases such as diabetes and heart disease. Experts believe this rise in obesity is due to lack of physical activity and an increase in the amount of high fat and sugary foods available to teenagers. Staying

active and eating foods that are low in fat and sugar promote a healthy weight for teens. Before placing a child or teenager on a weight control plan their doctor should always be consulted.

Eating disorders

An eating disorder is an emotional and physical problem associated with an obsession with food, body weight or body shape and is seen in both girls and boys. The most common types of eating disorders are anorexia, bulimia and binge eating. Teenagers tend to be very conscious of appearances and may feel pressure to be thin or to look a certain way, leading to a fear of gaining weight and potentially to an eating disorder. Some symptoms of eating disorders:

⇨ significant and sudden weight loss (15% below the normal BMI which is between 18.5 and 25);
⇨ preoccupation with body weight;
⇨ continual dieting (although thin);
⇨ preoccupation with food, calories, nutrition, and/or cooking;
⇨ lack of menstrual periods;
⇨ preference to eat in isolation;
⇨ compulsive exercise;
⇨ binge eating;
⇨ frequent use of the bathroom after meals;

⇨ self-induced vomiting or laxative use to control weight;
⇨ depression;
⇨ social withdrawal.

For parents who suspect their teen has an eating disorder, trying to help a child who doesn't think they need help can be hard. Remember that it's not your job to diagnose your child – only a doctor can do that, but you can approach your child about your concerns in a loving, supportive and non-threatening way. Express your concerns, explain why you are concerned and get your child to a medical professional for an objective and accurate assessment of their condition. Teens who suspect their friends, siblings or they themselves have a problem with body image or eating habits should talk to a trusted adult.

Remember, there is help out there and for more information, contact:
The Eating Disorders Association
Web: http://www.b-eat.co.uk/Home
Tel: 08456 341414

⇨ The above information is reprinted with kind permission from Tesco. Visit www.tesco.com/health/ for more information on this and other related topics.

© Tesco

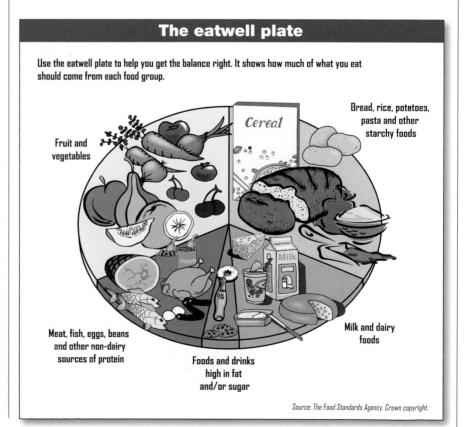

The eatwell plate

Use the eatwell plate to help you get the balance right. It shows how much of what you eat should come from each food group.

Fruit and vegetables

Bread, rice, potatoes, pasta and other starchy foods

Cereal

Milk

Meat, fish, eggs, beans and other non-dairy sources of protein

Foods and drinks high in fat and/or sugar

Milk and dairy foods

Source: The Food Standards Agency. Crown copyright.

Skin cancer now threatens women in their twenties

Information from Cancer Research UK

The deadliest form of skin cancer has now become the most common kind of cancer for women in their twenties – according to the latest figures from Cancer Research UK which launches its 2009 SunSmart campaign today.

Almost every day of the year in the UK a woman between 20 and 29 is diagnosed with malignant melanoma – the potentially fatal form of skin cancer. In this age range there are twice as many cases of melanoma as there are of breast cancer.

Latest figures show* around 340 women in their twenties were diagnosed with melanoma in a single year.

And for women in their thirties melanoma has risen to be the third most common cancer after breast and cervix.

Around 50 women under the age of 40 die from melanoma each year. Overall the disease kills around 1,800 people every year but rates are predicted to rise.

By the year 2024 Cancer Research UK statisticians predict that malignant melanoma will be the fourth most common cancer for men and for women – of all ages – rising from around 9,000 cases diagnosed each year now to more than 15,500.

Experts believe that binge tanning, usually on foreign holidays, and increasing use of sunbeds are prime reasons for the alarming rise in this life-threatening disease.

Caroline Cerny, Cancer Research UK's SunSmart campaign manager, said: 'Spending time on sunbeds is just as dangerous as staying out too long in sun. Sunbeds don't offer a safe way to tan. The intensity of UV rays in some sunbeds can be more than ten times stronger than the midday sun.

'Excessive exposure to UV damages the DNA in skin cells which increases the risk of skin cancer and makes skin age faster.

'But, importantly, if people take care not to burn in the sun and don't use sunbeds the majority of malignant melanoma could be prevented.'

A Cancer Research UK survey of 4,000 people last year revealed that one woman in three had used a sunbed. And research shows that using sunbeds under the age of 35 can increase the risk of melanoma by 75 per cent.

The survey also found that 80 per cent of sunbed users first used a sunbed under the age of 35.

A recent study found that nine per cent of 11- to 17-year-old girls have used a sunbed

---

Jenna Gurney, now 28, from London, was diagnosed with malignant melanoma when she was 21. She had used sunbeds twice a week since she was 16, regularly topping up her tan. A mole on her stomach got bigger and started to grow flaky so her GP advised it should be removed. She was shocked to be diagnosed with melanoma and had to endure an operation to remove her lymph nodes under her arms.

'When I was a teenager, my friends and I used sunbeds all the time. It was just so important to have a tan all year round and to top it up for nights out,' said Jenna, an administrator.

'When I used sunbeds I used an intensifier cream instead of any kind of protective sun lotion. On holiday I did put on sun lotion but never worried about regularly reapplying it or using a high factor.

'Even though the risks were at the back of my mind, I'm just one of those people who think it will never happen to me. If I could go back and have my time again I would never use sunbeds. I wouldn't want to go through the stress and worry of having cancer for the sake of a tan.

'I've always liked the look of a healthy glow but I am now really careful in the sun, stay in the shade and religiously apply sun lotion. Now I use fake tan products.

'It's only been since my cancer diagnosis that I understand the serious consequences of using sunbeds and spending too much time in the sun. I hope my story will make others aware of the risks of melanoma from using sunbeds.'

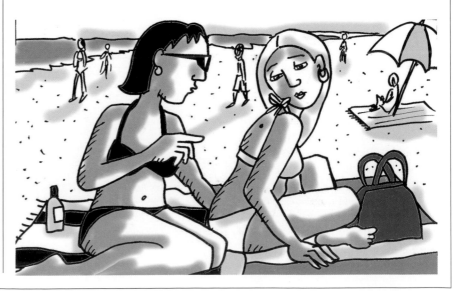

A recent study** found that nine per cent of 11- to 17-year-old girls have used a sunbed.

Sara Hiom, Cancer Research UK's director of health information, said: 'It is extremely worrying to see that so many young girls are using sunbeds. Young skin is delicate and so easily damaged by the sun. Damage from UV builds up over time. Every time young people use a sunbed they are harming their skin and increasing their risk of skin cancer.'

For more information on Cancer Research UK's SunSmart campaign visit www.sunsmart.org.uk. The SunSmart campaign is funded by the UK health departments.

Sunbeds and legislation

In Scotland legislation has been passed to ban under-18s from using sunbeds and for all sunbed salons to be supervised and proper information provided to customers. This has yet to be implemented. In England, Wales and Northern Ireland there is public concern about the issue but no existing plans for legislation.

Skin cancer facts

The most common kind of skin cancer is non-melanoma skin cancer. More than 75,000 cases are registered each year in the UK but it is estimated that the actual number is at least 100,000.

Around 9,000 cases of malignant melanoma are diagnosed each year in the UK. Incidence rates of this form of skin cancer have quadrupled since the 1970s. Around 2,000 people a year die from malignant melanoma.

Skin cancer: causes and risks

Excessive UV exposure is the main cause of both kinds of skin cancer. Other factors that increase skin cancer risk are:

⇨ People with light eyes or hair, who sunburn easily or do not tan;

⇨ People with a lot of moles, unusually shaped or large moles or a lot of freckles;

⇨ A history of sunburn doubles the risk of melanoma;

⇨ Using sunbeds;

⇨ Family history of skin cancer.

Finding skin cancer early saves lives.

Remember the SunSmart messages

Spend time in the shade between 11am and 3pm.

Make sure you never burn.

Aim to cover up with a t-shirt, hat and sunglasses.

Remember to take extra care with children.

Then use factor 15+ sunscreen.

Also report mole changes or unusual skin growths promptly to your doctor.

*Latest available figures from 2005
**Cancer Research UK and Department of Health study 2008
8 April 2009

⇨ The above information is reprinted with kind permission from Cancer Research UK. Visit www.cancerresearchuk.org for more.

© Cancer Research UK

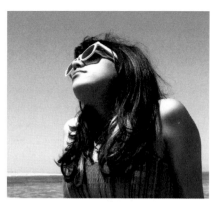

Young smokers fear future impact on their appearance

Information from the British Psychological Society

Young smokers say concern about the effects of smoking on their appearance is a good reason to quit smoking, but not until they see visible changes to their appearance. This is the finding of a study by Professor Sarah Grogan of the University of Staffordshire and colleagues Gary Fry, Brendan Gough and Mark Conner, published today (26 January 2009) in the *British Journal of Health Psychology*.

87 smokers and non-smokers aged 17-24 took part in the study, based on focus groups. The smokers discussed how smoking impacted negatively on physical appearance (skin, teeth, hair and weight), and how they made sense of their smoking. The non-smokers also discussed a potential link between appearance and smoking, together with any appearance-related concerns that would discourage them from taking up the habit.

Male and female smokers were concerned about the impact of smoking on their appearance, but would quit only if skin ageing, wrinkling or other negative effects on appearance became noticeable. The young people did not consider themselves at immediate risk of such effects as they were thought to occur in older smokers only. Non-smokers expressed concern about the impact on skin and teeth if they started smoking.

Professor Grogan said: 'Young adults have the highest rates of smoking in the UK; they are also likely to be concerned with their physical appearance. Emphasising the fact that skin damage caused by smoking may not be visible to the naked eye – but is still happening – might be an effective way to motivate young people to quit.'

The findings of this study will be used to inform anti-smoking campaigns targeted at young people.

'Our study suggests that campaigns that emphasise the negative effects that smoking can have on appearance are more likely to encourage young people to quit than those that focus on the impact of smoking on health,' Sarah concluded.

26 January 2009

⇨ The above information is reprinted with kind permission from the British Psychological Society. Visit www.bps.org.uk for more.

© British Psychological Society

Young people and smoking

Information from ASH

Smoking prevalence

Children become aware of cigarettes at an early age. Three out of four children are aware of cigarettes before they reach the age of five whether or not the parents smoke. Experimentation is an important predictor of future use: two out of three regular smokers say they started smoking before the age of 18. In 2008, 68% of pupils aged 11-15 said they had never tried smoking. This is higher than at any time since the young people's smoking survey began in 1982. The proportion of pupils who had tried smoking at least once (32%) represents a long-term decline since 1982, when 53% had tried smoking.

The annual Government survey of smoking among secondary school pupils defines regular smoking as smoking at least one cigarette a week. However, in 2008, pupils classified as regular smokers smoked a mean (average) of 39.3 cigarettes a week, approximately six a day. Occasional smokers smoked a mean of 3.9 cigarettes a week. These averages have remained at similar levels since 2004.

As in previous years, girls are more likely than boys to have ever smoked. This contrasts with the results of regional studies of children's smoking habits during the 1960s and 1970s

ash.
action on smoking and health

which showed that more boys smoked than girls and that boys started earlier. In 1982, at ASH's instigation, the government commissioned the first national survey of smoking among children and found that 11% of 11- to 16-year-olds were smoking regularly.

In 1998, the government set a target to reduce the prevalence of regular smoking among young people aged 11-15 from a baseline of 13% in 1996 to 11% by 2005 and 9% or less by 2010. The decline in smoking has been most marked among older pupils. The proportion of 14 year olds who smoked regularly fell from 13% in 2006 to 9% in 2008; among 15 year olds, 14% smoked regularly in 2008, compared with 20% in 2006.

What factors influence children to start smoking?

Children are more likely to smoke if one or both of their parents smoke and parents' approval or disapproval of the habit is also a critical factor. A Dutch study revealed that adolescents with both parents smoking were four times more likely to be a smoker

than their peers whose parents had never smoked. The same study also found that parental cessation when the children were young reduced the likelihood of adolescent smoking. Numerous studies have shown that most young smokers are also influenced by their friends' and older siblings' smoking habits. Other influences include tobacco advertising which fosters positive attitudes towards smoking and increases the likelihood of initiation. There is also a growing body of evidence suggesting that teenagers may also be influenced by viewing smoking in films.

Smoking, alcohol and drug use

There is a strong association between smoking and other substance use. The 2008 secondary school survey found that pupils who had taken drugs at least once in the previous year had more than 10 times the odds of being regular smokers compared with pupils who had never taken drugs. Similarly there is strong association between smoking and alcohol consumption, with the odds of being a regular smoker increasing with the number of units drunk in the previous week.

Smoking and children's health

Child and adolescent smoking causes serious risks to respiratory health, both in the short and long term. Children who smoke are two to six times more susceptible to coughs and increased phlegm, wheeziness and shortness of breath than those who do not smoke. Smoking impairs lung growth and initiates premature lung function decline which may lead to an increased risk of chronic obstructive lung disease later in life. The earlier children become regular smokers and persist in the habit as adults, the greater the risk of developing lung cancer or heart disease. Smokers are also less fit than non-smokers: the performance in a half marathon of a smoker of 20 cigarettes a day is that of a non-smoker 12 years older.

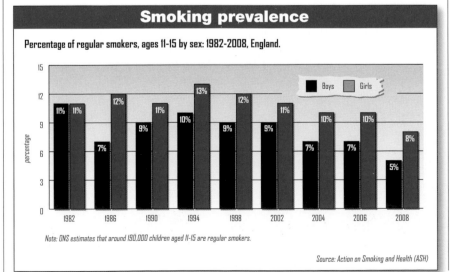

Smoking prevalence

Percentage of regular smokers, ages 11-15 by sex: 1982-2008, England.

Note: ONS estimates that around 190,000 children aged 11-15 are regular smokers.

Source: Action on Smoking and Health (ASH)

Children are also more susceptible to the effects of passive smoking. Parental smoking is the main determinant of exposure in non-smoking children. Although levels of exposure in the home have declined in the UK in recent years, children living in the poorest households have the highest levels of exposure as measured by cotinine, a marker for nicotine.

Bronchitis, pneumonia, asthma and other chronic respiratory illnesses are significantly more common in infants and children who have one or two smoking parents. Children of parents who smoke during the child's early life run a higher risk of cancer in adulthood and the larger the number of smokers in a household, the greater the cancer risk to non-smokers in the family. For more information see the ASH Research Report: *Passive smoking: the impact on children.*

Addiction

Children who experiment with cigarettes can quickly become addicted to the nicotine in tobacco. Children may show signs of addiction within four weeks of starting to smoke and before they commence daily smoking. One US study found that smoking just one cigarette in early childhood doubled the chance of a teenager becoming a regular smoker by the age of 17 and a London study suggests that smoking a single cigarette is a risk indicator for children to become regular smokers up to three years later. In the 2008 survey of schoolchildren in England, 69% of smokers aged 11-15 reported that they would find it difficult to go without smoking for a week while 76% thought they would find it difficult to give up altogether. During periods of abstinence, young people experience withdrawal symptoms similar to the kind experienced by adult smokers.

Smoking prevention

Since the 1970s, health education (including information about the health effects of smoking) has been included in the curricula of most primary and secondary schools in Great Britain. Research suggests that knowledge about smoking is a necessary component of anti-smoking campaigns but by itself does not affect

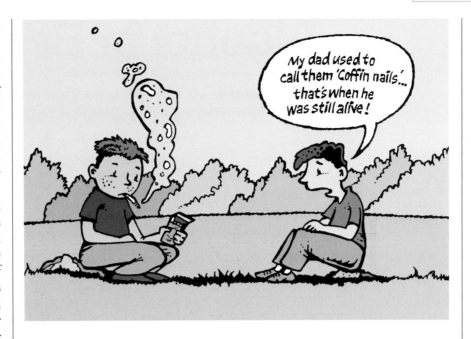

smoking rates. It may, however, result in a postponement of initiation. High prices can deter children from smoking, since young people do not possess a large disposable income: studies suggest young people may be up to three to four times more price sensitive than adults. In Canada, when cigarette prices were raised dramatically in the 1980s and the early 1990s youth consumption of tobacco plummeted by 60%. An American study has shown that while price does not appear to affect initial experimentation of smoking, it is an important tool in reducing youth smoking once the habit has become established.

Children, smoking and the law

On 1 October 2007, the legal age for the purchase of tobacco in England and Wales was raised from 16 to 18. The amendment was designed to make it more difficult for teenagers to obtain cigarettes, since, despite the law, children still succeed in buying tobacco from shops and vending machines. In 2008, the first time data were collected after the change in the law, 39% of pupils who smoked said they found it difficult to buy cigarettes from shops, an increase of 15% from 24% in 2006. There has also been a drop in the proportion of regular smokers who usually buy their cigarettes from a shop: from 78% in 2006 to 55% in 2008. The 2008 survey also found that 12% of 11- to 15-year-old regular smokers reported

that vending machines were their usual source of cigarettes, compared to 17% in 2006.

During 2006 there were 72 prosecutions in England and Wales for underage tobacco sales, with 59 defendants being found guilty. An amendment to the Criminal Justice and Immigration Act includes banning orders for retailers who persistently sell tobacco to persons under the age of 18. These measures came into force in April 2009.

Following a Government consultation on the future of tobacco control the Government has published a Health Bill incorporating measures to protect children and young people from smoking. These include tighter controls on the sale of cigarettes from vending machines and a ban on the display of tobacco at the point of sale.

Legislation alone is not sufficient to prevent tobacco sales to minors. Both enforcement and community policies may improve compliance by retailers but the impact on underage smoking prevalence using these approaches alone may still be small. Successful efforts to limit underage access to tobacco require a combination of approaches that tackle the problem comprehensively.

August 2009

⇨ The above information is reprinted with kind permission from ASH. Visit www.ash.org.uk for more information or to view references for this article.

© ASH

Alcohol in Britain

Trends show young men are binge-drinking less, but women are binge-drinking more

Research released today (6 May 2009) shows that the proportion of women who binge-drink almost doubled between 1998 and 2006 and is now at 15% (men who binge-drink increased by 1% to 23%). However, the proportion of 16- to 24-year-old men binge-drinking decreased by 9% since 2000. Researchers also found that whilst fewer children are drinking, those that do drink are drinking much more than they did in the past.

'Young men's drinking, including binge-drinking, has gone down in recent years, while middle aged and older people's drinking has increased'

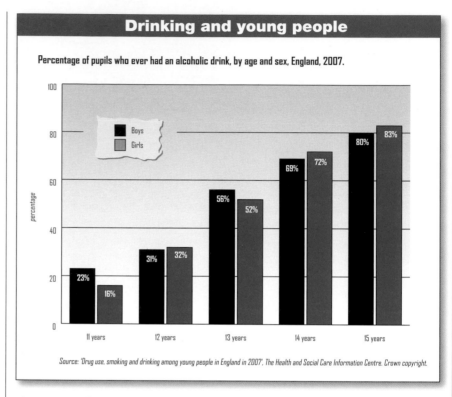

Drinking and young people

Percentage of pupils who ever had an alcoholic drink, by age and sex, England, 2007.

- Boys
- Girls

	11 years	12 years	13 years	14 years	15 years
Boys	23%	31%	56%	69%	80%
Girls	16%	32%	52%	72%	83%

Source: 'Drug use, smoking and drinking among young people in England in 2007', The Health and Social Care Information Centre. Crown copyright.

The research, carried out by a team from Oxford Brookes University for the Joseph Rowntree Foundation, looked at existing evidence on drinking trends in the general population over the last 20 to 30 years. Five trends highlighted in the report are:

An increase in drinking amongst women

In the UK, women are less likely than men to drink, and women who do drink consume less than men. However, the gender gap has generally narrowed over the last 15 to 20 years. Researchers suggest this might relate to the influence of advertising and also women's increased financial security and independence.

An increase in drinking among middle-age and older groups

In recent years there has been a steady increase in alcohol consumption in these age groups. Researchers say it is likely to be wealthier individuals who are drinking more; however, the report points out that alcohol is 65% more affordable now than in 1980.

A recent decrease in drinking among 16 to 24 year olds (both sexes but especially men)

The researchers were surprised to find that young adults are drinking less, especially in the face of rising consumption in the older age groups. Whilst this downturn might seem counter-intuitive, given the media attention on binge-drinkers, recent trends do indicate that this age group are not drinking quite as much as they once were.

An increase in alcohol consumption amongst children

Fewer children are drinking, but those that do drink are drinking much more than they did in the past. Researchers found that the most compelling consideration when trying to explain the rising trend in consumption amongst 11 to 13 year olds compared with older teenagers and young adults is the influence of parents, family, friends and the home environment.

An increase in drinking in Northern Ireland compared with the rest of the UK

Researchers found excessive weekly drinking has increased in Northern Ireland compared with Great Britain as a whole. One possible explanation for this is the change in licensing laws in 1996, and the rapid growth in the leisure industry since the peace process began.

Lesley Smith, the report's lead author, said: 'Much concern has been expressed in recent years about young people's drinking – and young people binge-drinking in particular. Many people will be surprised to learn that young men's drinking, including binge-drinking, has gone down in recent years, while middle aged and older people's drinking has increased.'
6 May 2009

⇨ The above press release is reprinted with kind permission from the Joseph Rowntree Foundation, the independent development and social research charity. Visit www.jrf.org.uk for more information.

© Joseph Rowntree Foundation

Binge drinking

Britain is known for its binge drinking culture, but do you know what effect it's having on your health?

What is binge drinking?

People drink for all sorts of reasons, mostly because in moderation alcohol helps you relax and feel more sociable. Binge drinking is all about boozing simply to get drunk.

There are many different definitions of binge drinking, and they tend to be a bit vague. A recent government report describes binge drinking as 'the consumption of excessive amounts of alcohol within a limited time period', which can mean different things to different people. Another commonly used definition is 'the consumption of twice the daily benchmark given in the Government's guidelines'. This equates to six to eight units for men and four to six units for women in one sitting.

How do I know how many units I'm drinking?

Here are some rough examples of how many units are in typical drinks:

⇨ Half a pint of beer or cider = 1.5 units;

⇨ A small glass (125ml) of wine = 1.5 units;

⇨ A single measure of spirits (e.g. whisky, vodka, rum or gin) = one unit.

The number of units can vary according to the brand of drink and whether you're male or female. For a more accurate picture check out Drink Aware's unit calculator and add up all the units you've drunk this week.

Give me the stats

Are you sure? They don't exactly paint a pretty picture. According to the Institute of Alcohol Studies, young people in the UK are the third worst binge drinkers in the EU. What's more, the Joseph Rowntree Foundation found that over 50% of 15 to 16 year olds have participated in binge drinking, and another report showed that 44% of 18 to 24 year olds are regular binge drinkers.

But I like getting lashed

Only you can take responsibility for your relationship with drink. It's just worth being aware of the impact binge drinking can have on your life.

Accidents happen

Statistically-speaking, if you're completely wasted you're more likely to harm yourself by falling into bushes or stepping out into moving traffic. Drunken drivers are another clear hazard, especially if you've gone along for the ride, and as alcohol affects judgement you may well agree to something you'd never do sober. It's estimated that alcohol features in 20-30% of accidents, and if you're comprehensively slaughtered from a holiday binge session then obviously things are more likely to go wrong for you.

Crime time

Binge drinking can bring you into contact with crime in several ways, as a victim or villain. For example, 76,000 facial injuries in the UK each year are linked to drunken violence. Alcohol is a major factor in 33% of burglaries and 50% of street crime. In short, you're vulnerable when smashed, and not in full control of your judgement, whether you're swinging a punch because you're plastered or getting decked by someone more drunk than you.

Bad skin

A heavy session can cause dehydration, which means your skin can miss out on a supply of vital nutrients.

Increased blood pressure and heart rate

Binge drinking on a regular basis can cause heart problems with your ticker later in life.

Liver problems

Alcohol in the body is processed by your liver. A heavy session places a big strain on this vital organ, and if you make it a regular date you run an increased risk of a disease called cirrhosis, in which liver cells turn to scar tissue. It may not seem like a big

deal now, but if the disease goes too far there is no cure.

Foot in mouth problems

Heavy drinking messes with your coordination, not just physically but speech-wise, too. Getting seriously drunk might give you the Dutch courage to make a move at the office party, but consider what kind of result you can hope to achieve in that condition. Slurring your words isn't much of a turn on, while statistics suggest one in five binge drinkers who do pull regret it afterwards.

Binge behaviour

Binge boozing on a regular basis can shape your future drinking habits, often leading to a harmful relationship with alcohol.

⇨ The above information is reprinted with kind permission from TheSite. Visit www.thesite.org for more information.

© *TheSite*

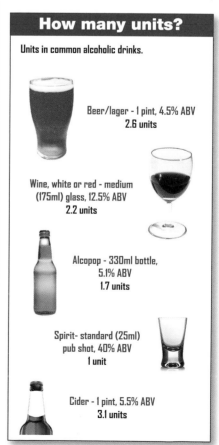

How many units?

Units in common alcoholic drinks.

Beer/lager - 1 pint, 4.5% ABV
2.6 units

Wine, white or red - medium (175ml) glass, 12.5% ABV
2.2 units

Alcopop - 330ml bottle, 5.1% ABV
1.7 units

Spirit- standard (25ml) pub shot, 40% ABV
1 unit

Cider - 1 pint, 5.5% ABV
3.1 units

Britain's 'chronic' teenage binge-drinking problem

Britain's 'chronic' teenage binge-drinking problem has been highlighted by another European poll

The survey of 35 countries found the UK had the third highest number of 15 and 16 year olds with an alcohol problem. Professor Martin Plant, the University of the West of England academic who led the research, said: 'The UK retains its unenviable position in relation to both binge-drinking, intoxication and alcohol-related problems among teenagers.

'This problem is both serious and chronic. I hope that the Government will prioritise policies that are effective to reduce heavy drinking and alcohol-related disorder and health problems among young people.'

This is the most detailed international study carried out into binge-drinking and drug use among teenagers.

It included a sample of 1,004 boys and 1,175 girls from the UK, who were also found to suffer from high levels of relationship, sexual and delinquency problems.

The survey found that more than half of British teenagers had been binge-drinking in the past month, but girls were more likely to drink to excess than boys.

A statement from the university said: 'The fact that some teenage girls are binge-drinking even more than boys suggests that in the UK and elsewhere a profound social change has been taking place.

'It is clearly no longer socially unacceptable for females to drink heavily or to become intoxicated.

'This may reflect factors such as greater female social and economic empowerment and changing social roles as well as the marketing practices of the beverage alcohol industry.'

The UK had the third-highest number of 15 and 16 year olds with an alcohol problem

Only youngsters in Bulgaria and the Isle of Man abused drink to a greater extent.

But the report found the number of teenage smokers in the UK had fallen since 1999, whilst only 11% of British teenagers admitted to smoking cannabis in the past month.

Professor Plant added that many teenagers in the UK were developing serious health problems and dying prematurely because of their drinking.

He said: 'There is a clear scientific consensus that alcohol education and mass media campaigns have a very poor track record in influencing drinking habits.

'Far more effective – and cost effective – policies include using taxation to make alcohol less affordable.

'Many people whose alcohol consumption is generally moderate also experience some adverse effects from their drinking.

'It is therefore recommended that a minimum price of 50p per unit of alcohol should be introduced. This would save over 3,000 lives per year.

'It would also reduce problems such as absenteeism, public disorder and hospital admissions. This measure would particularly affect harmful and hazardous drinkers.

'It could save £1 billion per year in the cost of alcohol-related harm.'
26 March 2009

© *Telegraph Media Group Limited (2009)*

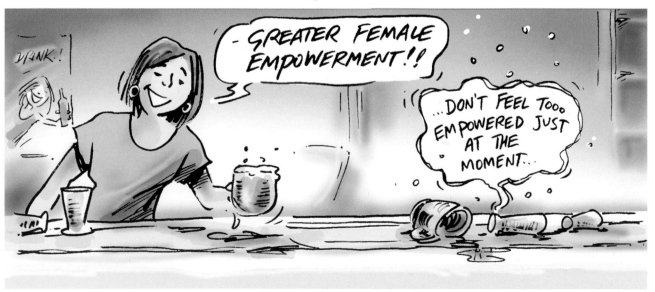

Underage drinking debate

Underage drinking is one of the problematic issues constantly associated with adolescence. Eshe Nelson, 17, speaks to her peers and gives their perspective on the debate as well as her own

Everyone knows that drinking alcohol under 18 is illegal, and just as many of us know that it's a law liberally broken. Because of this the drinking behaviour of young people is widely criticised, and although some people may have provoked damning media reports of reckless drunken behaviour, for the majority of young people there is very little justice in these accusations.

According to most young people, the adult perception of what teenagers actually get up to on a Friday night is far from real

It's understandable that underage drinking is considered a serious problem, but it's also fair to say that it's a problem which is exaggerated by the national media, leading some adults into condemning its hellish ways. However, according to most young people, the adult perception of what teenagers actually get up to on a Friday night is far from real.

Young people I spoke to agreed. Hannah Austin, 19, reflected back on when she was underage and said: 'I think adults can't relate to the culture. My parents don't really understand why me and my friends got drunk before we went out – to save money.' Ellie describes underage drinking as: 'part of growing up, something you try with your friends for the first time'.

Adults being misguided by the media and rarely being a first hand witness has led to an often unrealistic image. Melissa Freeman, 17, says that adults think underage drinking 'is worse than it is and that every teenager is paralytic every night'. Popular British comedy, *Skins*, has played a part in creating this image. Initially praised for being so true-to-life of the average British teenager, the infamous Skins Party* now represents what adults consider a typical teenage party. Annabel Davis, 19, thinks that *Skins* is 'really unrealistic, you may go to one party like that in your life but it's not like that every single weekend'.

Between the demands of school, work and trying to get enough sleep, there is very little time to socialise during the week and no one wants to experience a Sunday morning headache on a Thursday half way through Maths class.

Although the majority of young people do drink and the responsible attitude doesn't extend to everyone, a lot of young people don't consider always getting drunk an idealistic way of life. Melissa Freeman condemns binge drinking as; 'a lack of self-control and thinking it's cool to be throwing up and passing out'. Underage drinking is recognised as being 'unhealthy' and Ellie Child, 17, described the situation as 'out of hand' because teenagers are starting to drink younger and younger. Selina Purcell, 17, also recognises the dangers of drinking: 'Everyone knows it's dangerous because the effects of it won't kick in until we're older, we ignore it and drink excessively regardless.'

The government's bid to control what is being considered a worsening epidemic is apparently failing miserably. Legal consequences of underage drinking include arrest and fines of up to £500; however, the majority of government legislation targets license holders and does very little to discourage underage drinking. According to Selina, 'underage drinkers are so common, the age limit doesn't seem to have a major effect on who is drinking, it just stops people drinking in certain places'. Hannah agrees with this, stating: 'it might discourage places not to sell it to underage people but we were never worried about getting caught drinking underage'. The laws against drinking seem to be having the opposite to their intended effect. Annabel described it as 'like wanting the forbidden fruit you can't have' and if Eve couldn't fight the temptation, what hope does anyone have.

Everyone needs to find things out for themselves and make their own mistakes. Young people need

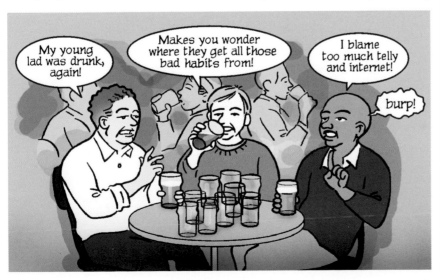

to experiment with alcohol, act excessively and learn their limits. The novelty then quickly wears off and young people can drink fully aware of what they're doing and by the time they're legally adults they can behave responsibly when the responsibilities start to pile up.

So maybe the answer is to accept that underage drinking happens, then it would stand more chance of being tackled effectively, rather than people either assuming young people are horrendous binge drinkers or ignoring the problem because it's illegal.

Drinking is dangerous to everyone's health so rather than having one rule for some and another for others, maybe it's time for adults to lead by example

---

And maybe in trying to find a solution we should take a closer look at why young people start binge drinking in the first place. The UK has the third highest rate of binge drinking in Europe and according to the Institute of Alcohol Studies (IAS), young people drink because it's become an integral part of their social scene. Well the IAS is right and this tradition didn't start with 16 year olds in 2009. It should come as no surprise that the drinking habits of adults have rubbed off on young people. According to Melissa, adults 'still drink too much on average and just ignore any mention of livers'. Drinking is dangerous to everyone's health so rather than having one rule for some and another for others, maybe it's time for adults to lead by example.

A Skins Party involves loads of people, alcohol, drugs, strobe lights and dance music.

This article was written by Eshe Nelson, 17.

⇨ This story was produced by Headliners, a journalism programme for young people aged 8 to 19. www.headliners.org

© Headliners

More young people seek help for problems with drugs

Information from the National Treatment Agency

Figures published today by the National Treatment Agency (NTA) for BBC Radio 1 have shown that more people than ever under the age of 30 are getting help for problems with drugs. The NTA says the rise is due in large part to an expansion in drug treatment over the last few years, meaning that if you have a drug problem you are now much more likely to get the help you need. Although the numbers of people accessing drug treatment is increasing, there is little reliable evidence to say that use is becoming more widespread amongst young people.

Key findings from the NTA figures show that:

⇨ The main drugs those aged 13-18 are being treated for are alcohol and/or cannabis; for 19-24 year olds it is heroin/opiates followed by cannabis and then cocaine; and for 25-30 year olds, heroin/opiates are the most common substances people in that age range are being treated for.

⇨ Addiction to Class A drugs is rare amongst under-18 year olds in particular. Of the 23,905 under-18s being treated for substance misuse in England in 2007/08, just over 1,600 were for heroin/opiates (3%), cocaine (3%) and crack (less than 1%) as the main drug misuse and they received specialist treatment support.

⇨ There is a marked increase in the number of 19 to 24 year olds being treated for cocaine, which then decreases for the 25- to 30-year-old age group. The NTA believes the most likely explanation is that this reflects patterns of drug use.

Tom Aldridge, NTA Young Persons Manager, said:

'We had an enormous increase in the number of young people coming into treatment, which is more to do with drug services being more available and increased investment. But what is clear is that there is more of a focus on cannabis, alcohol and cocaine powder use, and it's a very small minority that are using crack cocaine and opiates.

'Now any young person who needs help is much more likely to get it, and will be treated whatever the substance or substances they are misusing.'

For 2006-07, there was improved and increased reporting by service providers to the National Drug Treatment Monitoring System, which may account for some of the rise.
8 June 2009

⇨ The above information is reprinted with kind permission from the National Treatment Agency for Substance Misuse. Visit www.nta.nhs.uk for more information.

© NTA

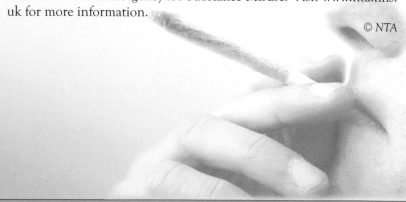

Drug problems

If you're worried about your own drug taking, or know someone who is abusing or misusing drugs, it's good to know the facts

Why take drugs?

Drug users don't start using drugs with the intention of becoming addicted. But with many drugs containing substances that are addictive, people who use them casually in their spare time can then become dependent on needing to use them regularly.

Reasons why people start using drugs can include:

➪ to escape problems they may be having in other parts of their life;

➪ peer pressure and fitting in with another group of people;

➪ being curious about the effects of drugs.

If you start to use drugs on a regular basis, or if you become dependent on them, it can affect your family and friends as well as having a serious impact on your own physical and mental well-being.

Drug overdoses can be fatal, and you can die instantly from misusing drugs that you can buy over the counter – this includes things like aerosols, glues and other solvents.

Drug overdoses can be fatal, and you can die instantly from misusing drugs that you can buy over the counter

Signs of drug abuse and misuse

There is not a common list of symptoms that you can use to tell if you or someone you know is misusing drugs. That's because drug use affects different people in different ways depending on the type of drugs they're using.

Although anxiety, tiredness and a change in sleeping habits can also be signs of drug use, they can also be caused by changes in your body, stress or other problems.

Drugs and the law

Drugs are categorised into three classes based on their overall level of harm; Class A drugs being the most dangerous, and Class C drugs being less dangerous. However, all the drugs in all three classes are harmful and are addictive.

Remember that all drugs are illegal, even Class C drugs like GHB and ketamine. If you're caught selling them on to other people, or carrying a small amount of drugs in your pocket, it's likely that the police will get involved. If you're found guilty of any of these offences, you may face a fine or time in custody, with Class A drugs carrying the most severe sentences.

Worried about a friend?

If you suspect that one of your friends or relatives is abusing drugs, you may want to approach them and talk about it.

It's not your responsibility to make them stop, but you can tell them about how their behaviour is affecting your relationship with them.

If they come to you asking for help with their problems, then it's important to listen and help them find the right information and treatment.

Talk to FRANK

If you're worried about drug abuse and addiction, the Talk to FRANK helpline can help.

FRANK runs a free helpline and a website that explains how different types of drugs can affect you. You can get confidential advice by calling 0800 77 66 00, seven days a week. Calls are free and they won't show up on your phone bill, but you may be charged if you use a mobile.

➪ The above information is re-printed with kind permission from Directgov. Visit www.direct.gov.uk for more information.

© Crown copyright

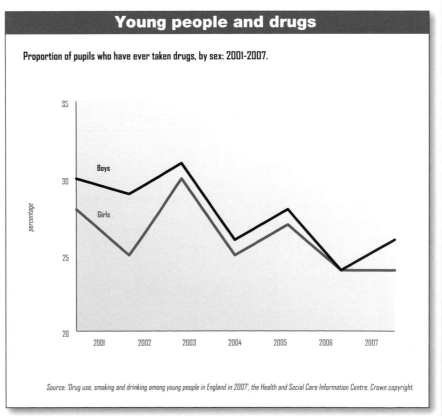

Young people and drugs

Proportion of pupils who have ever taken drugs, by sex: 2001-2007.

Source: 'Drug use, smoking and drinking among young people in England in 2007', the Health and Social Care Information Centre. Crown copyright.

Acne

Acne usually starts in puberty, although it affects adults, too. Around 80% of teenagers get some form of acne, and there are many myths around what causes it. Here are the facts and details of treatments

Acne consists of spots and painful bumps on the skin. It's most noticeable on the face, but can also appear on the back, shoulders and buttocks. Severe acne can cause scarring.

So what causes acne? It's mostly because of the way skin reacts to hormonal changes. The skin contains sebaceous glands that naturally release sebum, an oily substance that helps protect it. During puberty, raised levels of the hormone testosterone can cause too much sebum to be produced. This happens in both boys and girls.

The sebum can block hair follicles and when dead skin cells mix with the blockage, this can lead to the formation of spots. Bacteria in the skin multiply, which can cause pain and swelling beneath the blockages.

There are different kinds of spots:
- Blackheads. Small, blocked pores.
- Whiteheads. Small, hard bumps with a white centre.
- Pustules. Spots with a lot of pus visible.
- Nodules. These are hard, painful lumps under the skin.

Inflammatory acne is when the skin is also red and swollen, and this needs to be treated early in order to help prevent scarring.

Picking or squeezing spots can cause inflammation and lead to scarring. Spots will eventually go away on their own, but may leave redness in the skin for some weeks or months afterwards.

Acne can become worse during times of stress, and in women can be affected by the menstrual cycle.

If you have acne, wash your skin gently with a mild cleanser and use an oil-free moisturiser. Scrubbing or exfoliating can irritate the skin, making it look and feel sore.

Myths

Many people say that eating chocolate or greasy foods causes acne, but this isn't true. Acne isn't caused by bad diet.

Indy Rahil of the British Skin Foundation says: 'Your diet does not cause spots or acne. But if you have a pre-existing skin condition, including acne, some people might find that certain foods make the condition worse.' If you notice that your acne does gets worse if you eat a certain food, avoid eating it.

Some people believe that acne is caused by bad personal hygiene, but this is not true. If you are going to get acne, you will get it no matter how much you clean your skin. Too much cleaning can make the condition worse by removing the protective oils in your skin.

Treatments

Acne will usually go away on its own, but it can take many years. There are treatments that can help clear acne more quickly. Over-the-counter treatments can help with mild acne. Ask a pharmacist to advise you on which treatment might help, and how long you will have to use it for. You might not see results for several weeks.

If over-the-counter treatments don't help, there are treatments available on prescription. Your GP can assess how bad your acne is and discuss the options with you.

Mild, non-inflammatory acne consists of whiteheads and blackheads. Treatment includes gels or lotions that can contain retinoids (vitamin A), adapalene to slow the growth of skin cells, or benzoyl peroxide, which is antibacterial.

Mild-to-moderate inflammatory acne has some pustules and nodules. Treatment can include gels with benzoyl peroxide or azelaic acid (which stops the growth of bacteria), antibiotic creams or oral antibiotics. It can take up to eight weeks before you see a difference in your skin, and treatment might need to be continued for six months.

In women, contraceptive pills that contain oestrogen can help clear acne.

If acne is severe, your GP can refer you to a dermatologist who can prescribe medication to reduce sebum production.

There are light and laser therapies that claim to help get rid of acne, but few, if any, of these are available on the NHS.

- The above information is reprinted with kind permission from the NHS. Visit www.nhs.uk for more information on this and other related topics.

© Crown copyright

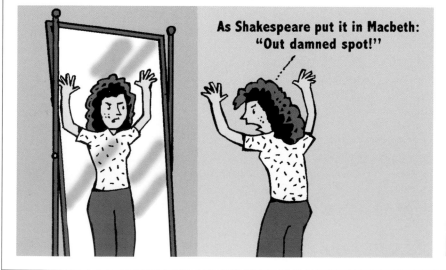

As Shakespeare put it in Macbeth: "Out damned spot!"

Am I ready for sex?

Information from AVERT

This is a question that almost everyone will ask themselves at some point in their lives, but unfortunately not many people will be able to answer it with a definite 'yes' or 'no'.

Having sex for the first time can be a very special experience, but it can also lead to all sorts of complications. Sex without a condom or other form of contraception can result in pregnancy, and if your partner has HIV or a sexually transmitted infection (and you might not always know they do), you can become infected too. There can also be emotional consequences to having sex with someone – it can really change a relationship, and not always for the better. Sex can be enjoyable with the right person, but it's very easy to make mistakes and end up hurt, which is why people advise you: 'don't have sex until you're ready!'

It takes more than just being a legal age to make you ready for sex – you need to be emotionally ready too

---

Of course it's all very well saying this, but how do you know when you're ready? Legally, you aren't allowed to have sex with anyone until you're over the age of consent. But it takes more than just being a legal age to make you ready for sex – you need to be emotionally ready too.

We obviously don't know you, so you're the only person who can truly judge if you're ready to have sex. But we can suggest some questions that will hopefully help you to work it out:

1) Are you doing this because YOU want to?

Or are you thinking about having sex because someone else wants you to? Maybe you're not sure you're ready, but your partner is keen? Or perhaps there's a bit of 'peer pressure' – all your friends seem to be having sex, so you feel you should be too?

Do any of the following sound familiar?

⇨ 'You would if you loved me!'
⇨ 'It's only natural!'
⇨ 'Everyone else is doing it!'
⇨ 'Don't you want to make our relationship stronger?'
⇨ 'You'll have to do it sometime – why not now, with me?'
⇨ 'I'll be gentle, and it'll be really great, I promise!'
⇨ 'I'll only put it in for a second...'

If you recognise any of these phrases, then you should think carefully! These are not the right reasons to have sex. A partner who says things like this is probably trying to put pressure on you and might not really care whether you're ready or not – this person doesn't respect your feelings, and they're probably not the right person to have sex with.

Nor should you have sex just because your friends are saying things like:

⇨ 'You mean you've never done it?!?'
⇨ 'I lost it when I was 12...'
⇨ 'Yeah, I've had sex loads of times...'
⇨ 'You're a virgin, you wouldn't understand...'
⇨ 'No-one'll be interested in you if they hear you're frigid.'
⇨ 'It's amazing – you don't know what you're missing!'

It may feel like your friends are all more experienced and knowledgeable, but we guarantee they're probably not! Many of them will only be saying this sort of thing because they think everyone will laugh at them if they admit they've never really done anything! Besides, being sexually experienced at a young age doesn't necessarily make someone mature or sensible – in fact, it usually indicates the opposite.

2) Do I know my partner well enough?

If you've only just met your partner, haven't been going out with them very long, or perhaps don't even really know them, then sex is never going to be a really good experience because there won't be much trust between you. If you've never even kissed the person you're with, then you're definitely not ready to have sex with them!

Sex can leave you feeling very vulnerable afterwards in a way you might not be prepared for, so it's better to be with someone that you know is likely to be sticking around. Usually, you'll have better sex with someone you know really well, are comfortable with, and who you can talk to openly about relationships and feelings. Sex will be best with someone you love.

3) Is it legal?

The age of consent differs between countries. In most states of the U.S., for instance, it ranges between 16 and 18. In the UK and India it's 16. In Spain, it's 13 while in some Muslim countries, sex is illegal unless you're married. Have a look at the age of consent page on the AVERT website (www.avert.org) to find out exactly what it is where you live.

So why do countries have a legal age for having sex? Because this is the age when the government believes young people are mature enough to handle the responsibilities that come with having sex. All too often people think they are ready when they're not.

Age of consent laws are also designed to prevent older people from taking advantage of children and young teenagers who may not understand the consequences of having sex, or even what sex is.

4) Do I feel comfortable enough with my partner to do this, and to do it sober?

It's natural to feel a little embarrassed and awkward the first time you have sex with someone because it's not something you've ever done before. Your boyfriend or girlfriend will probably feel the same. But if you don't trust your partner enough not to laugh at you or you don't feel you can tell them you've never had sex before, then it's far better to wait until you can.

And if you think you'll have to drink a lot of alcohol before you do it so you feel relaxed enough, or you only find yourself thinking about having sex when you're drunk, then that suggests you're not ready. A lot of people lose their virginity when they're drunk or on drugs, and then regret it. So if you're worried that you're going to be in a situation where you might be tempted to do something you wouldn't do normally, restrict your drinking, keep off the drugs, or make sure you stick with a sober friend who can look after you! Have a look at the 'drink, drugs and sex' page on the AVERT website (www.avert.org) for more information.

5) Do I know enough about sex?

Do you know what happens during sex? Do you know how it works, what it's for and how and why a woman can get pregnant? Do you know about sexually transmitted infections? Lots of people worry that they're going to make a fool of themselves or do something wrong. Well, you shouldn't have to worry if you're with a partner who cares about you - (s)he won't laugh. And if you're not with a partner who cares, you probably shouldn't be doing it! Physically, sex is actually quite simple, but the more you know, the more comfortable you'll feel. Have a look at the teens' pages on the AVERT website for more information.

6) Will I be glad when I'm older that I lost my virginity at the age I am now?

Imagine that you're looking back at yourself in ten years' time. What do you think you'll think then about how and when you lost your virginity? Is there any way in which you might regret it? The answer should be 'no' – if it's not, you're probably not yet ready for sex.

7) Can I talk to my partner about this easily?

If you can't talk about sex, then you're not ready to have sex. It's as simple as that. Being honest about how you're feeling will make it easier for both of you, and will make sex better in the future.

8) Do I know how to have sex safely?

It's really important that you know how to protect against pregnancy, STIs and HIV. Again, this is something you need to talk to your boyfriend or girlfriend about before the event, so you're both okay about what you're going to use. Have a look on the teens' contraception options page on the AVERT website for more details.

Especially with things like condoms, it's good to have a bit of practice putting them on, and to feel okay about doing it - it's not enough just to get a condom if you're not confident enough to use it - they're no good if they stay in your pocket the whole time!

9) Do we both want to do this?

You may decide that you are ready to have sex, but it might be that your partner isn't, even if they have had sexual partners before. For sex to work, you both have to be willing to do it. Don't ever pressure anyone to have sex if they're not sure - this is very wrong, and it'll cost you your partner's respect and the respect of other people.

Also - there's a fine line between pressuring someone to have sex and forcing someone to have sex - if you put too much pressure on someone, it can become force - and if you force someone into sex, you can be prosecuted for rape.

10) Does sex fit in with my/ their personal beliefs?

It may be that you, your partner or your family have beliefs that say sex at a young age (or before marriage) is wrong. Do you feel comfortable going against these views? Will it cause you unnecessary worry and guilt if you do (or frustration and heartbreak if you don't!)? Some young people will have sex simply because their family has banned them from doing so, even if they don't realise that this is the reason. Having sex as an act of rebellion may feel great at the time, but if anything goes wrong, you face a very difficult situation, as you may not be able to rely on your family's support.

Even if everything goes well, keeping sex (and all the emotions that go with it) a secret can be very hard – so, if possible, you should make sure you have someone else to talk to that you can trust to keep it to themselves. But remember, the decision to have sex should be an agreement between you and your partner, and while other people may help or influence your decision, they shouldn't make it for you.

So, how did you do? If you answered 'Yes!' to all ten of these questions, then you're probably pretty much ready, as long as BOTH of you feel okay about it.

If you didn't, then there are probably some issues you need to work through first, because all of these questions are important.

First-time sex is always going to be scary whatever age you are when you have it. It can sometimes seem like losing your virginity is the most important thing in the world. But you can't get your virginity back once it's gone, so what is really important is that you have enough respect for yourself to wait until you're truly ready, and can truly trust the person you're with.

Good luck, have fun, and stay safe!

⇨ The above information is reprinted with kind permission from AVERT. Visit www.avert.org for more information on this and related topics.

© AVERT

Healthy sex life

You can have healthy and safe sex by taking control and managing your sex life in a way that fulfils both you and your partner

A healthy sex life can mean a variety of things. The most important thing is that it's your sex life we're talking about. So that means finding out what makes you comfortable, and what works for you.

It might be that this varies over time and it can depend on many things. Sometimes your sex life is busy and other times it's less of a priority, but either way it can still be a healthy sex life.

It's all about you taking control and managing your situation. Hopefully that will produce a result that fulfils both you and your partners.

What you can do
Here are some strategies to help you manage your sex life:
⇨ get regular checkups;
⇨ keep up-to-date on sexual health matters;
⇨ take action if you notice anything out of the ordinary;
⇨ get help with sexual problems or dysfunctions;
⇨ talk to your partner.

Your sex life is going to change as time passes, just as other aspects of your life do. A bit of thought means that your sex life can contribute to the rest of your life rather than detracting from it.

Checkups
If you go to your local genito-urinary medicine (GUM) clinic you can get a regular free checkup for sexually transmitted infections (STIs). You might be able get this service from your doctor (GP) but GUM clinics will protect your confidentiality (you can even remain anonymous, although if you do give your name this information won't be passed onto any other agencies).

Having regular checkups means that you'll have a clear picture of your sexual health. So not only will you be able to relax, but you'll be in a better position to talk to your partners.

Keeping up-to-date
It's sensible to keep up-to-date on sexual health matters. After all, things do change: while some issues might be less of a worry now than they were in the past, you should be aware of any new infections and how they may affect your sex life. You can get this information at your GUM clinic or online.

Most STIs can be cured with no lasting effect to your health if they are dealt with early enough and if you follow the medication instructions

---

Take action
If you notice anything unusual about your sexual health, get it checked. Most STIs can be cured with no lasting effect to your health if they are dealt with early enough and if you follow the medication instructions.

If your symptoms seem trivial or embarrassing, then you could call a sexual health helpline and get some initial advice over the phone.

Sexual dysfunction
Similarly, if you're suffering from a sexual problem or dysfunction it might be worth getting some help. A lot of these problems have a biological basis and can be treated successfully.

It could be that you're suffering for nothing. The professionals who deal with these things have often dealt with similar cases as that's what they do every day. You can find out more from the Sexual Dysfunction Association.

Talk to your partner
Communication with your partner is vital. What kind of safer sex measures would they rather take? What do you prefer?

Not everyone feels comfortable disclosing everything about their sexual health. Safer sex means that this shouldn't be a problem. If you have different ideas then try to reach a compromise that makes you both feel comfortable.

⇨ The above information is reprinted with kind permission from the Terrence Higgins Trust. Visit www.tht.org.uk for more information.
© Terrence Higgins Trust

STD diagnoses

STD diagnoses at GUM (genito-urinary medicine) clinics in the UK: 1998-2007.

Year	Syphilis (primary and secondary)	Gonorrhea (uncomplicated)	Chlamydia (uncomplicated)	Herpes (first attack)	Genital warts (first attack)	All new diagnoses
1998	139	13,212	48,726	17,248	70,291	244,282
1999	223	16,470	56,991	17,509	71,748	261,406
2000	342	21,800	68,332	17,823	71,317	284,035
2001	753	23,705	76,515	18,944	73,458	303,169
2002	1,257	25,591	87,588	19,438	74,969	324,170
2003	1,652	24,073	96,150	19,233	76,599	346,168
2004	2,283	22,326	104,739	19,073	80,059	363,289
2005	2,721	19,248	109,418	19,830	81,201	368,258
2006	2,684	18,898	113,783	21,797	83,624	375,843
2007	2,680	18,710	121,986	26,062	89,838	397,990
% change (2006-2007)	0%	-1%	7%	20%	7%	6%
% change (1998-2007)	1,828%	42%	150%	51%	28%	63%

Source: 'All new episodes seen at GUM clinics: 1998-2007. United Kingdom and country-specific tables'. Health Protection Agency, July 2008.

Sexually transmitted infections

Information from Brook

First things first

Sexually transmitted infections (STIs) are a major cause of ill health. They can also cause ectopic pregnancy (where an egg is fertilised and becomes implanted in the fallopian tube), and may also lead to infertility in both men and women.

Since 1995 there have been large increases in the number of people diagnosed with STIs, particularly women in their late teens and men in their early twenties. This may be because people are more aware of STIs and are visiting clinics to be tested.

What are the symptoms?

Symptoms vary between STIs and some have no symptoms at all. Where there are symptoms, these may include unusual discharge from the vagina or penis, heavy periods or bleeding between periods, pain or burning sensation when passing urine, rashes, itching or tingling around the genitals or anus.

Tests and treatment

Most STIs can be easily diagnosed and treated at genito-urinary medicine (GUM) clinics, which are usually based in local hospitals. If you think you may have an STI, you can refer yourself to any GUM clinic for advice and treatment. The service is completely confidential and you don't have to go to your nearest clinic if you don't want to.

Contact our Ask Brook service to find a GUM clinic. Or look in the phone book under GUM or sexual health.

Tests for STIs vary. Some involve taking swabs from the cervix or tip of the penis. Others involve taking a blood sample.

Before being tested it is usual to see a health adviser who will discuss safer sex with you so that you can avoid infections in the future. Counselling is usually offered before testing for HIV so that you are prepared for the implications of the test result if it is positive.

If you test positive for any STI, the clinic will encourage you to talk to your current partner and, where relevant, previous partners, so that they can also be tested. If you prefer, the clinic can do this for you without revealing your identity. Most STIs are treatable with antibiotics.

Avoiding STIs

STIs are usually passed on by sex with an infected person, though some can be passed on in other ways as well. They can be caught during oral, vaginal or anal sex.

Using a male or female condom every time you have sex will stop the transmission of most STIs. Condoms can be used in addition to another method of contraception, such as the pill, which does not protect against infections. This is often referred to as the 'double dutch' method.

Dental dams (small squares of latex) can also be used as a barrier during sex involving contact between the mouth and the vagina, or the mouth and the anus.

Condoms are easily available from Brook Centres (for under-25s) and family planning clinics, and dental dams are available from GUM clinics.

Types of STI

There are 25 types of sexually transmitted infection. Some can be acquired without sexual contact. The most common infections are:
⇨ Chlamydia;
⇨ Gonorrhoea;
⇨ Genital herpes;
⇨ Genital warts;
⇨ Non-specific genital infections (NSGIs);
⇨ HIV and AIDS;
⇨ Hepatitis B;
⇨ Trichomoniasis;
⇨ Syphilis.

The following are not necessarily transmitted through sexual contact:
⇨ Candidiasis (thrush);
⇨ Pubic lice;
⇨ Scabies.

⇨ The above information is reprinted with kind permission from Brook. Visit www.brook.org.uk for more.

© Brook

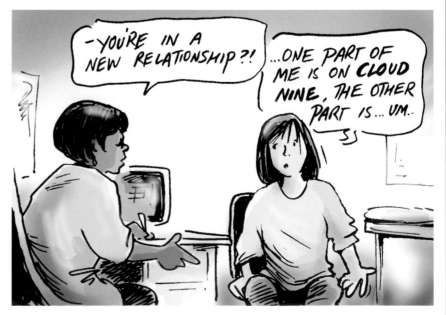

Sex secrets putting young people's health at risk

Young people are putting each other's sexual health at risk because they are too embarrassed to tell their partner they have a sexually transmitted infection (STI)

A new NHS survey shows that 16% of under-25s would not tell the person that they are sleeping with if they found out they had the STI chlamydia, while 19% are 'not sure'.

16% of under-25s would not tell the person that they are sleeping with if they found out they had the STI chlamydia

---

However, chlamydia has serious health consequences. Left untreated, chlamydia can prevent both men and women from being able to have children and lead to other health problems such as arthritis. Yet the NHS poll shows nearly a quarter (24%) of under-25s would not tell their previous sexual partners that they had chlamydia, even if they thought they were at risk of infection.

Men were much more likely to stay silent about the infection than

If caught early, chlamydia can be easily treated with one dose of antibiotics

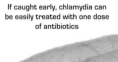

women. 21% would not tell the person that they are currently sleeping with, while 21% said that they weren't sure. Over a quarter (29%) said they would not tell a previous sexual partner if they were at risk of being infected (compared to 19% of women).

The survey is published to coincide with MAYbe month, the start of a new NHS campaign to combat the spread of chlamydia, the most prevalent and fastest growing STI among under-25-year-olds. Throughout May, the boroughs of Kensington & Chelsea, Hammersmith and Fulham & Westminster have been holding an intensive chlamydia screening drive and information campaign to ensure that people get tested and treated for chlamydia.

Chris Morgan of Westside Contraceptive Services, who supply screening services to the NHS, says: 'Anyone who has ever had unprotected sex, including oral sex, can have chlamydia. It usually does not have any symptoms, so it is very difficult to know if you or the person you are sleeping with has it. As the survey shows, you can't always rely on your partner to be honest with you about their sexual health. The only way to be sure that you don't have chlamydia is to get tested.

'The test for Chlamydia is quick, easy and confidential. One urine sample shows if you've got chlamydia and it can be easily treated with one dose of antibiotics. If you are aged 16-24 and live in West London you can get a free test by post, from your GP or participating pharmacists or from

Westside Contraceptive Services' clinics. Find out more at www.check-kit.org.uk'

Despite being physically intimate, under-25s appear to be shy when it comes to talking about their sexual health. The majority (64%) of under-25s who had unprotected sex in the last six months did not ask the person that they were sleeping with about their sexual history. Almost half (47%) of men and women surveyed also admitted that embarrassment was the main reason they would not tell their partner they had chlamydia.

Chris Morgan continues: 'Embarrassment is not an excuse to put another person's health at risk. chlamydia can have severe health consequences if it is left untreated, stopping both men and women from having children and causing arthritis.'

Around one in ten people aged under 25 who are tested for it have chlamydia

---

Around one in ten people aged under 25 who are tested for it have chlamydia. The National Chlamydia Screening Programme recommends that all sexually active young people have a chlamydia test every year or when they change sexual partners, regardless of whether they have any signs or symptoms.
21 May 2009

⇨ The above information is reprinted with kind permission from Westminster PCT. Visit www.westminster-pct.nhs.uk for more.
© *Westminster PCT*

STIs and young people

Information from the Health Protection Agency

Messages to be used with young people

All those interested in the sexual health of sexually active young people should use their particular communication skills to relay the following key messages for the prevention of STIs:

⇨ Have fewer sexual partners and avoid overlapping sexual relationships.

⇨ Use a condom when having sex with a new partner and continue to do so until both have been screened.

⇨ Get screened for chlamydia every year and whenever you have a new partner.

⇨ If you are a man who has sex with men, then always use a condom and have an annual sexual health screen, including an HIV test.

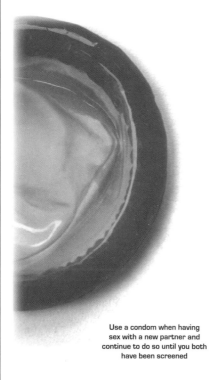

Use a condom when having sex with a new partner and continue to do so until you both have been screened

Sexually transmitted infections (STIs), including HIV, remain one of the most important causes of illness due to infectious disease among young people (aged between 16 and 24 years old). If left untreated, many STIs can lead to long-term fertility problems (e.g. with chlamydia or gonorrhoea). Infection with HIV or the strains of human papillomavirus (HPV) that cause cervical cancer can lead to long-term illness and possible death.

Key findings

⇨ Young people (aged 16-24 years old) are the age group most at risk of being diagnosed with a sexually transmitted infection, accounting for 65% of all chlamydia, 50% of genital warts and 50% of gonorrhoea infections diagnosed in genitourinary medicine clinics across the UK in 2007.

The most common sexually transmitted infection in young people is genital chlamydia

---

⇨ The most common sexually transmitted infection in young people is genital chlamydia. The National Chlamydia Screening Programme in England performed 270,729 screens in under 25 year olds in 2007: 9.5% of screens in women and 8.4% in men were positive for chlamydia. A further 79,557 diagnoses of genital chlamydia infection were made among young people in genitourinary medicine clinics in the UK in 2007 (a rate of 1,102 per 100,000 16-24 year olds), a rise of 7% on 2006.

⇨ Genital warts were the second most commonly diagnosed sexually transmitted infection among young people in genitourinary medicine clinics, with 49,250 cases diagnosed in 2007 (682 per 100,000), an 8% rise on 2006.

⇨ In 2007, 702 young people were diagnosed with HIV, representing 11% of all new HIV diagnoses. Young men who have sex with men remain the group of young people most at risk of acquiring HIV in the UK.

⇨ Increases in diagnoses reflect greater ascertainment of cases through more testing and improved diagnostic methods, as well as indicating increased unsafe sexual behaviour among young people.

Recommendations

⇨ There should be easy access for young people to sexual health services that can provide advice, screening and treatment of STIs including HIV.

⇨ Interventions to promote sexual health among young people should be designed from a strong evidence base and evaluated for their continuing effectiveness.

⇨ The delivery of high quality personal, relationship and sexual health education, which should include sexuality among its themes, is essential in providing young people with the necessary information and skills to be able to negotiate and engage in safer sexual behaviour.

⇨ Information from the new improved STI surveillance will enable primary care organisations to better target future prevention efforts, especially in vulnerable populations such as men who have sex with men and ethnic minority communities with the highest rates of STIs.

July 2008

⇨ The above information is reprinted with kind permission from the Health Protection Agency. Visit www.hpa.org.uk for more information on this and other related topics.

© HPA

Contraception – the facts

When you start thinking about contraception there's a lot of information to take in. It's confusing at first, but getting to know the facts can help you look after yourself and make smart choices

Essential protection

Contraception can prevent unplanned pregnancy. Most young people choose the pill or condoms as they are safe and easy-to-use options.

There are lots of other contraception types to choose from, including diaphragms, hormone injections, implants, IUS, IUD and sterilisation. The best contraception for you depends on your age and individual circumstances, so it's best to go and chat to your doctor or visit a young person's clinic to find out what will suit you best.

Your best protection is to use a condom. Not just sometimes, but every time you have sex

---

Condoms rule

When you use condoms properly they can prevent pregnancy and, unlike all the other methods of contraception, they protect you against STIs too.

Safer sex means making sure you don't catch a sexually transmitted infection (STI). Your best protection is to use a condom. Not just sometimes, but every time you have sex.

The pill

The contraceptive pill is a tiny tablet women can take every day to stop them getting pregnant.

You can get the pill from a doctor or local family planning clinic for free. It is almost 100% effective in stopping pregnancy as long it's taken properly - but it won't protect you from picking up an STI.

Emergency contraception pills

If you've had sex without using contraception, or you think your contraception hasn't worked, you can use emergency contraception. If you act quickly, this can usually prevent pregnancy. Emergency contraception pills (also called 'morning after' pills) should be started within 72 hours from the time you had unprotected sex. They are much more effective if you take them within 24 hours, so it's important to act quickly.

Going to the clinic

You can get free contraception at a contraception clinic, including free condoms. You can also get emergency contraception and pregnancy tests. If you are pregnant, there will be someone there you can talk to.

Even if you're under 16, you have the same right to confidentiality as everyone else. You don't have to give your real name and your GP is only contacted with your permission – you can tick a box to say no.

Safer sex – why bother?

You might think there's no point in safer sex, especially if your boyfriend or girlfriend has promised they don't sleep around. But people don't always tell the truth — and even if they are faithful, if they had sex with someone before you, you're still at risk of getting an STI.

One in nine people has had an STI so the chances of catching something are higher than you might think. And because some infections don't have obvious symptoms (some have no symptoms at all) you can never know for sure if the person you are sleeping with has one. The best protection against STIs is to use a condom every time you have sex – even if you're taking the pill. It won't spoil your fun and it could save your life.

Research shows that 40% of first visits to sex advice services by young women were to get emergency contraception.*

There is no law that stops people under the age of 16 buying condoms, and no law restricting the seller.
*Source: Brook, Young people's sex advice services; delays, triggers and contraceptive use, Brook Publications, 2000.

⇨ The above information is reprinted with kind permission from r u thinking?. Visit www.ruthinking.co.uk for more information.

© r u thinking?

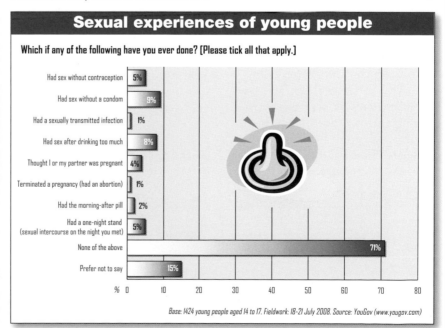

Sexual experiences of young people

Which if any of the following have you ever done? [Please tick all that apply.]

	%
Had sex without contraception	5%
Had sex without a condom	9%
Had a sexually transmitted infection	1%
Had sex after drinking too much	8%
Thought I or my partner was pregnant	4%
Terminated a pregnancy (had an abortion)	1%
Had the morning-after pill	2%
Had a one-night stand (sexual intercourse on the night you met)	5%
None of the above	71%
Prefer not to say	15%

% 0 10 20 30 40 50 60 70 80

Base: 1424 young people aged 14 to 17. Fieldwork: 18-21 July 2008. Source: YouGov (www.yougov.com)

Concern over young people's risky sex

Sexual health survey shows HIV/AIDS awareness in decline among 16 to 24 year olds, while fewer use condoms

75% of sexually active youngsters are not using condoms, says the Staying Alive Foundation survey.

Awareness of the dangers of HIV/AIDS is decreasing among young people at a time when fewer are practising safe sex, a survey has revealed.

Nearly 60% of 16 to 24 year olds questioned thought they were not at risk of contracting the infection after having unprotected sex and 8% believed taking a contraceptive pill offered protection against infection.

75% of sexually active youngsters are not using condoms

Almost 14% thought the fact that they were not gay ensured they could not contract HIV/AIDS while another 13% said they were either too young to be affected or felt 'perfectly healthy'.

The newly released results have emerged from a survey commissioned in spring of 2,550 young people on behalf of the Staying Alive Foundation charity, which is supported by MTV UK and The Body Shop. The most notable finding, that 75% of 16 to 24 year olds are not using condoms, has already been published.

These latest figures show that on average young people admit to having had an average of 6.81 sexual partners, and to having had unprotected sex with an average of 3.44 partners.

More than 35%, however, said they had been tested for HIV. Of those who had not, 16% said they did not know where to go to get tested, 5% were too scared of the outcome and 7% were too embarrassed.

Broken down by region, youngsters in Leeds appear to be the most reckless – the number having unprotected sex there is 86%. In Manchester, around 70% think they have 'no chance' of contracting the virus.

More than 35% of those questioned could not recall ever having seen an advertising campaign about HIV/AIDS. The findings echo concerns among medical charities that many young people are unaware of the dangers.

The Department of Health last year estimated that 73,000 are living with HIV in the UK, one third of whom did not know they were infected. Knowledge about safe sex practices also appears to be declining. In 2007, 79% of people said they knew HIV could be passed on by sex between a man and woman without a condom; in 2000, the figure was 12% higher.

Georgia Arnold, the official in charge of social responsibility at MTV, said: 'Young people do not remember the government campaigns of the 1980s and generally aren't responding to the current safe sex campaigns. Without that awareness young people are lulled into a false sense of security – they think the risks have gone away when in fact they are as real as ever.'

She was disappointed that two £8,000 grants for work on HIV/AIDS awareness offered by the organisation's charitable Staying Alive Foundation had not been claimed in the UK this year. The lack of applications, she feared, reflected lower awareness of the dangers and a mistaken belief that the disease is cureable. Other results from the survey show that more men – nearly a quarter – think women run the most risk of contracting HIV/AIDS. Only 10% of women think the same.

4 June 2009

© Guardian News & Media Ltd 2009

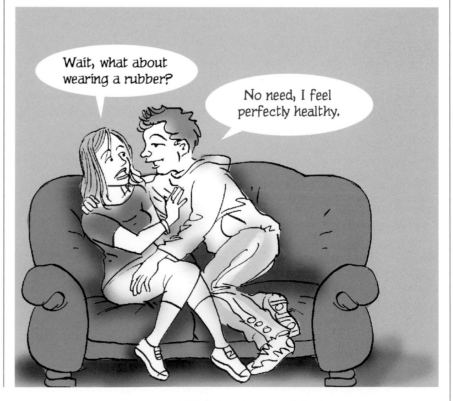

Children and young people

Information from the Mental Health Foundation

The emotional wellbeing of children and young people is just as important as their physical health. Most children grow up mentally healthy, but certain risk factors make some more likely to experience problems than others.

Children and young people's negative feelings usually pass. If further help is needed, a range of professionals can offer support, usually through school or on the NHS.

Advice for young people

If you are in distress, you are not alone. One in five young people experience a mental health problem in the course of a year. You may find it helpful to talk to a friend, your boyfriend or girlfriend or a relative about your problems if you do not want to speak to a parent. Or you may prefer to talk to someone else you trust like a teacher or faith leader.

You can seek help on your own by ringing a confidential helpline or by seeing a professional, but if you are under 16 a parent/carer's consent is usually needed before you can get any medical care. You have a right to privacy if you do not want to tell anyone about your conversations with professionals.

Good mental health

The emotional wellbeing of children is just as important as their physical health. Good mental health allows children and young people to develop the resilience to cope with whatever life throws at them and grow into well-rounded, healthy adults.

Things that can help keep children and young people mentally well include:

⇨ being in good physical health, eating a balanced diet and getting regular exercise;

⇨ having time and the freedom to play, indoors and outdoors;

⇨ being part of a family that gets along well most of the time;

⇨ going to a school that looks after the wellbeing of all its pupils;

⇨ taking part in local activities for young people.

Other factors are also important, including:

⇨ feeling loved, trusted, understood, valued and safe;

⇨ being interested in life and having opportunities to enjoy themselves;

⇨ being hopeful and optimistic;

⇨ being able to learn and having opportunities to succeed;

⇨ accepting who they are and recognising what they are good at;

⇨ having a sense of belonging in their family, school and community;

⇨ feeling they have some control over their own life;

⇨ having the strength to cope when something is wrong (resilience) and the ability to solve problems.

Most children grow up mentally healthy, but evidence suggests that more children and young people have problems with their mental health today than 30 years ago. That's probably because of changes to the experience of growing up and to the way we live now.

Dealing with change

The things that happen to children won't usually lead to problems with their mental health on their own, but traumatic events can trigger problems for children and young people whose mental health is not already robust.

Changes often act as triggers: moving home or school or the arrival of a new brother or sister, for example. Some children who start school feel excited about making new friends and doing new activities, but there may also be some who feel anxious about entering a new environment.

Teenagers often experience emotional turmoil as their minds and bodies develop. An important part of growing up is working out and accepting who you are. Some young people find it hard to cope and may experiment with alcohol, drugs or other substances that can alter how they feel.

Risk factors

There are certain 'risk factors' that make some children and young people more likely to experience problems than other children, but they don't necessarily mean difficulties are bound to come up or are even probable.

Some of these factors include:

⇨ having a long-term physical illness;

⇨ having a parent who has had mental health problems, problems with alcohol or has been in trouble with the law;

⇨ experiencing the death of someone close to them;

⇨ having parents who separate or divorce;

⇨ having been severely bullied or physically or sexually abused;

⇨ living in poverty or being homeless;

⇨ experiencing discrimination, perhaps because of their race, sexuality or religion;

⇨ acting as a carer for a relative, taking on adult responsibilities;

⇨ having long-standing educational difficulties.

How parents can help

If parents have a warm, open relationship with their children, their children will usually feel able to tell them if they are troubled. One of the most important ways to help is to listen to them and take their feelings seriously. They may want a hug, they may want you to help them change something themselves or they may want practical help.

Children and young people's negative feelings usually pass. However, it's a good idea to get help if your child is distressed for a long time, their negative feelings are stopping them from getting on with their lives, their distress is disrupting family life or they are repeatedly behaving in ways you would not expect at their age.

Whatever life brings is a booklet for parents and carers which outlines the things that keep children and young people in good mental health and suggests what can help when children are troubled.

Types of mental health problems

If your child has been diagnosed with a particular mental health problem, you may find it useful to find out more in our booklet *Whatever life brings*.

Some of the mental health problems that can affect children and young people are listed below.

Depression affects more children and young people today than in the last few decades, but it is still more common in adults. Teenagers are more likely to experience depression than young children who rarely face depression.

Self-harm is a very common problem among young people. It describes the different ways that people deliberately harm their bodies, to help them deal with intense emotional pain.

Children and young people with a **generalised anxiety disorder** become extremely worried. Very young children or children starting or moving school may have separation anxiety.

Post-traumatic stress disorder can follow physical or sexual abuse, witnessing something extremely frightening, being the victim of violence or severe bullying or living through a disaster.

Children who are consistently overactive ('hyperactive'), behave impulsively and have difficulty paying attention may have **Attention Deficit Hyperactivity Disorder (ADHD)**. Many more boys than girls are affected, but the cause of ADHD isn't fully understood.

Eating disorders usually start in the teenage years and are more common in girls than boys. The number of young people who develop an eating disorder is small, but eating disorders such as anorexia nervosa and bulimia nervosa can have serious consequences for their physical health.

Professional help

If your child is having problems at school, a teacher, school nurse, school counsellor or educational psychologist may get in touch with you. Otherwise, go to your GP or speak to a health visitor. These professionals are able to refer a child to further help. Different professionals often work together in Child and Adolescent Mental Health Services (CAMHS).

Most support for children and young people who are troubled is provided free by the NHS, your child's school or your local council's social services department. In some parts of the country, there are long waiting lists for children and young people to see mental health specialists or to have a talking therapy on the NHS. Some people choose to pay for their children to have treatment.

Talking it through

Assessing and treating children and young people with mental health problems isn't the same as for other health problems. There is more emphasis on talking and on understanding the problem to work out the best way to tackle it. For young children, this may be done through playing.

Most of the time, the action that professionals recommend is not complex and it often involves the rest of the family. Your child may be referred to a specialist who is trained to help them explore their feelings and behaviour. This kind of treatment is called a talking therapy, psychological therapy or counselling.

Medication

More research has concentrated on

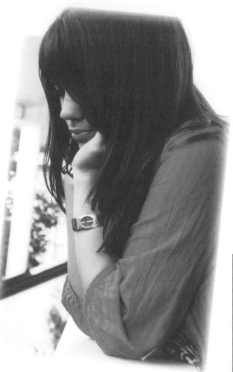

the effect on adults of drugs for mental health problems than on children. Children and young people need to be assessed by a specialist before they are prescribed any drugs. There is a lot of evidence that talking therapies can be effective for children and young people, but drugs may be also be important in some cases.

Confidentiality

The professionals supporting your child will keep information about them and your family confidential. Young people can seek help on their own, either by ringing a helpline or by approaching a professional directly, but your consent is usually needed for them to get medical care if they are under 16. Young people have a right to privacy if they do not want to talk to you about their conversations with professionals, but you should still respond sensitively if they seem to be upset.

Written in 2008
Statistics taken from The Fundamental Facts, *the Mental Health Foundation's digest of mental health facts and figures.*

⇨ The above information is reprinted with kind permission from the Mental Health Foundation. Visit www.mentalhealth.org.uk for more information.

© *Mental Health Foundation*

Young people's mental health ignorance

Information from Great Ormond Street Hospital for Children NHS Trust (GOSH)

⇨ GOSH launches new mental health section for teenagers on it's general health information resource for young people, Children First for Health. Visit http://www.childrenfirst. nhs.uk/teens/health/mental_ health/

⇨ Almost half (46 per cent) of 12-18 year olds in the UK cannot name a single mental health condition;

⇨ Less than half (47 per cent) think schools do enough to raise awareness of mental health issues and nearly half (43 per cent) don't think or don't know if there is enough information available for people their age;

⇨ There are clear discrepancies in views held by boys and girls on most common mental health conditions among young people;

⇨ 37 per cent of 12 to 18 year olds would turn to Internet first for mental health advice;

⇨ Nico Mirallegro, who plays *Hollyoaks*' schizophrenic character Newt, supports launch of new website.

Almost half (46 per cent) of 12-18 year olds in the UK cannot name a single mental health condition, new research has revealed.

Boys aged 12-14 are least likely to be able to name a mental health condition, almost two-thirds (59 per cent), according to the poll conducted by Great Ormond Street Hospital for Children NHS Trust (GOSH). Young people, of both genders, also incorrectly labelled Down's syndrome and dyslexia as mental health-related conditions.

Less than half of those polled (47 per cent) agreed that schools were doing enough to raise awareness of the subject, and nearly half (43 per cent) don't believe or don't know if there is enough information available on mental health issues for people their age.

1.4 per cent of 11-16 year olds in Great Britain are said to be 'seriously depressed'

Children First for Health, a GOSH website for children, young people and families with health-related concerns, has launched a new interactive mental health section aimed at 12-18 year olds. It includes clinically approved mental health condition factsheets, treatments and therapies, drug information, general mental health and well-being advice and articles on life on an adolescent ward. Audio podcasts of young people's first-hand accounts of life on an in-patient psychiatric ward and dealing with different mental health conditions, including eating disorders and drug addiction, are also featured.

The Populus poll also showed substance abuse (31 per cent), depression (16 per cent) and self-harm (15 per cent) are considered the most common mental health problems among young people, but there were clear discrepancies in the views held by boys and girls, and those falling into different age brackets.

Anorexia was identified by nearly one-fifth (19 per cent) of girls aged 12-18 as the second most common mental health problem among people their age, while for 17 per cent of boys it was depression. For girls aged 12-14 anorexia is considered the joint first most common mental health condition (26 per cent) with substance abuse. For boys in the same age bracket anorexia was named joint fourth most prevalent with phobias (nine per cent), with substance abuse considered most common (35 per cent).

1.4 per cent of 11-16 year olds in Great Britain are said to be 'seriously depressed', and between 1 in 12 and 1 in 15 children and young people deliberately self-harm, with over 25,000 admitted to hospital each year due to the severity of their injuries.

Dr Jon Goldin, consultant child and adolescent psychiatrist at GOSH said: 'For too long now there has been a stigma attached to living with a mental health condition. It is important that young people feel they can come forward and speak out if they or someone they know is experiencing mental health difficulties. The crux of the matter is that these conditions are quite treatable and there is no shame in seeking help for them.

'Our research shows that many teenagers feel there is not enough information on mental health conditions available to them, and with so many unable to name a mental health condition, the launch of the new section of Children First for Health website is crucial to our work in trying to address this. It has been designed specifically to appeal to 12-18 year olds, as well as health professionals, teachers and support organisations working with young people, providing them with guidance and advice as well as audio stories from other young people living with mental health conditions and what helps them to feel better.'

Girls aged 17-18 are the most likely group to gather mental health knowledge from celebrities, with half (50 per cent) agreeing with the statement 'famous people who talk about problems like these have given me a greater understanding of the subject'.

Hollyoaks' Nico Mirallegro, whose character Newt has been diagnosed with Schizophrenia, is supporting the launch of the new section.

Nico said: 'I think for many people my age there is a lot of confusion around the subject of mental health. Some will have a condition without even realising it. For many, confiding in family or friends will be difficult as they might feel ashamed or embarrassed. A resource like this is brilliant for young people, and being online allows them to gather information in their own time and in a private way if that is what they choose to do.'

With 37 per cent of 12-18 year olds saying they turn to the Internet first for advice on mental health issues, these findings support the need for a trusted resource like this

Marcella McEvoy, Children First for Health project manager, added: 'Our own analysis of 4,000 online anonymous enquiries shows that psychosocial enquiries are the most popular topic requests. With 37 per cent of 12-18 year olds saying they turn to the Internet first for advice on mental health issues, these findings support the need for a trusted resource like this, which aims to demystify this complex subject area, and signpost users to further sources of specialist support and treatment.'

To broaden the site's visual appeal it has been designed in the style of three different notebooks, allowing users to click into the book of their choice to view information.
7 September 2008

⇨ Reproduced with kind permission from Great Ormond Street Hospital for Children NHS Trust. Visit www.ich.ucl.ac.uk for more information.
© GOSH 2008

Depression among the young at alarming level

By Mary O'Hara

⇨ *Nearly half regularly feel stress, finds Prince's Trust.*
⇨ *Situation likely to worsen as recession takes hold.*

A significant number of young people are depressed or struggling to cope and the situation is likely to worsen as the recession takes hold, according to a report by the Prince's Trust. One in ten 16 to 25 year olds polled by the charity for its Youth Index study said they felt that life was meaningless, and more than a quarter (27%) said they were always or often down or depressed. Almost half of all those surveyed (47%) said they were regularly stressed.

The trust, which interviewed more than 2,000 young people across Britain, said the results were 'alarming'. Young people not in work, training or education were worst affected, the research found.

Some 37% of those outside paid employment or education admitted to being frequently down or depressed, while 27% said their lives had no purpose. With young people expected to bear the brunt of job losses over the coming year, the findings are likely to raise concerns among policymakers.

Martina Milburn, chief executive of the Prince's Trust, said the study revealed 'an increasingly vulnerable generation'. Paul Brown, a director at the trust responsible for the research, added: 'We already have evidence that young people are likely to be disproportionately affected during a recession. We also know that young people often have problems, especially those without supportive families. That one in ten young people think their life is not worth living is a really worrying thing to see quantified.'

Brown said the Prince's Trust, which provides support to about 40,000 young people a year, is introducing a new mental health awareness programme for team leaders in local projects to identify early signs of distress.

Peter Kellner, of YouGov, which conducted the research, said the majority of young people had a generally positive outlook on life. He warned, however, that the serious concerns of the 'core' of unhappy people under the age of 25 'need to be addressed'. He added that failing to take the issue seriously 'would be storing up big problems for the future'.

Concerns about the mental health and wellbeing of young people have risen sharply following reports about the emotional fragility of the current generation of children and teenagers, and problems around violence and knife crime.

In April last year the Children's Society's Good Childhood Inquiry, a state-of-the-nation overview of childhood, said in an interim report that more than a quarter (27%) of the 8,000 14 to 16 year olds it interviewed regularly felt depressed. The inquiry, a two-year rolling programme of research, also reported that just 9% of adults felt children are happier today than when they were growing up.

The final report, by Lord Richard Layard, the economist and author of the book *Happiness*, is due to be published at the end of this month. The Prince's Trust research could raise additional concern because it suggests that the emotional malaise already identified by the Children's Society in younger teenagers is stretching into early adulthood.
5 January 2009

© *Guardian News & Media Ltd 2009*

One in five young people have self-harmed

Information from YouthNet

More than one in five 16 to 24 year olds (21%) have self harmed, according to the results of a survey launched today (Monday 2 March 2009) by youth mental health charity 42nd Street, youth homelessness charity Depaul UK and online communications charity YouthNet.

More than one in five 16 to 24 year olds (21%) have self harmed

---

The YouGov survey of over 2,000 people aged 16 and over also indicates that friends and family of people who self-harm may be giving well intentioned but potentially harmful advice, because of a poor understanding of the best ways to provide support.

Key survey findings include:

⇨ More than half (57%) of the 16 to 24 year olds surveyed knew someone who has self-harmed in the past;

⇨ 42% of 16 to 24 year olds surveyed agreed with the statement 'I am confident I could give good advice

to someone I discovered was self-harming';

⇨ However, a third (32%) of 16 to 24 year olds said that their first reaction to discovering that someone close to them was self-harming would be to ask them to stop – advice that experts say is understandable but could be counterproductive as it can place unrealistic emotional demands on the person;

⇨ Almost a third (30%) of respondents aged 25 and over agreed with the statement 'I am confident I could give good advice to someone I discovered was self-harming';

⇨ Almost one in five respondents aged 25 and over (18%) said that their first reaction on discovering someone close to them was self-harming, would be to ask them to stop.

The results come as the group of youth charities launch an awareness and marketing drive aimed at young people affected by self-harm, to raise awareness of the advice and information available on YouthNet's guide to life for 16 to 24 year olds, TheSite.org, at www.TheSite.org/selfharm.

Paul Marriot, Chief Executive of Depaul UK, says: 'A number of the young people we work with on a daily

basis are dealing with self-harm issues. Usually, young people who self-harm do so as a way of coping with complex and difficult situations and although it's understandable that a parent, friend or carer's instinct would be to try and stop the person from self-harming, it's actually the issues behind it that need addressing, not the physical aspect of what the person is doing to themselves.'

The online survey also found that few young people considered GPs as a source of information on the issue, with only one in ten young people surveyed (15%) saying that a medical professional would be the first place they would go to for advice about self-harm. However, 43% of this age group cited the Internet as their first port of call.

Over a third (38%) of respondents over the age of 25 said that they would go to 'a medical professional' for advice and information first.

Psychotherapist and TheSite.org self-harm expert and advisor, Andrea Scherzer, says: 'Traditional methods of accessing health information are losing favour with a younger generation who are used to gathering information online, anonymously and instantly.

'This is why it's essential that factual, accessible advice on mental health and self-harm is made available online, allowing young people affected, and those around them, to get a real understanding of the issues and the best way to provide and access support.'

The new self-harm resource (launched in January 2009) is hosted on YouthNet's guide to life for 16 to 24 year olds, TheSite.org (at www.TheSite.org/selfharm) and provides detailed information on the subject through podcasts, video, written articles, real-life stories and case studies. Young people can also

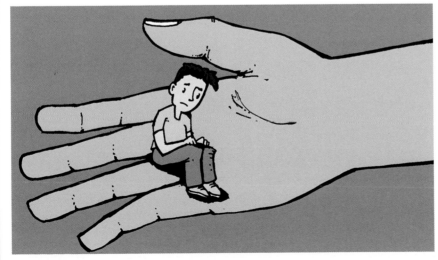

support, and gain support from, other young people through specialist discussion boards moderated by the charities. Professional advice is available via a confidential question and answer service and a series of live chats.

Vera Martins, Director of 42nd Street, says: 'Self-harm is a highly emotive issue and is often misunderstood. It is something that most people struggle to understand and talk about. Young people who self-harm are often perceived as "attention seekers" – we wish to challenge this kind of a stereotype and other myths connected to self-harm by raising awareness, creating an environment where people can talk about it openly and are aware of the help and support available.'

Anyone concerned about someone who is self-harming can follow TheSite. org's clear and simple advice:

⇨ Despite how distressed you might feel after having discovered or suspected your friend or relative is self-harming, try to focus on listening to them and what they are feeling and what kind of support they might need, rather than immediately reacting to the self-destructive behaviour itself;

⇨ Self-harm is a sign that something is wrong. It is usually a response to emotional distress and for some young people it is an important coping mechanism. So even if you feel shocked, try to speak with the person about your concerns in a calm and respectful way;

⇨ Don't make them promise not to do it again. A guilt trip won't help anyone. It can even make things worse, so try not to place emotional demands on them they probably won't be able to keep;

⇨ It's a positive step if someone has managed to open up to you, but getting help from a trained counsellor or health professional is important. Encourage them to seek specialist help and offer to go with them if they're worried about doing it alone. TheSite.org/ selfharm is a good first step;

⇨ Make sure you get support too – it is distressing for you too so make sure you get the help you need in order to support your friend or relative.

Visit www.TheSite.org/selfharm for more information or advice.
2 March 2009

⇨ The above information is reprinted with kind permission from YouthNet. Visit www.youthnet.org for more information.

© YouthNet

The epidemic of self-harm

Information from the Samaritans

Talk confidentially to Samaritans any time of the day or night. Whatever you're going through, whether it's big or small, don't bottle it up. We are here for you if you're worried about something, feel upset or confused, or just want to talk to someone.

Those aged between 11 and 25 years old are more likely to deliberately harm themselves

---

Binge-drinking and drug taking among young people are rarely out of the headlines, but one issue remains a taboo subject: self-harming. With recent figures reported by the *Independent on Sunday* and released in the Psychiatric Morbidity Survey revealing the increasing prevalence of self-harm, the lid is finally being lifted on the very real problem of those that deliberately hurt themselves to cope with feelings of distress.

The rise in self-harm

The number of people harming themselves deliberately has increased by a third in the past five years, according to new figures seen by the *Independent on Sunday*.

The newspaper revealed in March that there were 97,871 hospital admissions for deliberate self-harm in England in 2007-08 – 4,337 of them for children under the age of 14. Meanwhile, last month's annual Psychiatric Morbidity Survey revealed that nearly 12 per cent of women aged between 16 and 24 admitted to self-harm in 2007 – a rise of 80 per cent since 2000.

Speaking to the *Independent on Sunday*, Dr Andrew McCulloch, chief executive of the Mental Health Foundation, said: 'Self-harm is often a secret activity and people will avoid going to hospital if possible. So the fact we've seen such a substantial rise in hospital admissions is worrying and could be the tip of the iceberg.'

Why self-harm?

Figures show that those aged between 11 and 25 years old are more likely to deliberately harm themselves, with at least 1 in 15 young people having self-harmed in the UK, according to the Mental Health Foundation.

Self-harm not only damages the physical health of an individual, it can have far wider consequences, seriously affecting relationships with families and friends and having a detrimental impact on a person's wellbeing.

For many, self-harming acts as a coping mechanism, which enables a person to express difficult emotions, suggests the Mental Health Foundation. Those who hurt themselves deliberately often feel that physical pain is easier to deal with than the emotional pain they are experiencing. But, as mental health specialists warn, the behaviour only provides temporary relief and fails to deal with the underlying issues that a person is facing.

Highest levels in Europe

Although self-harming is most common among young people, a study undertaken by mental health charity SANE, published in December 2008, found that people of all ages are self-harming. Some participants of the study reported that they first started to harm themselves when they were as young as four; others had not started self-harming until they were in their late fifties.

Commenting on the research, chief executive Marjorie Wallace said: 'Over the last few years SANE has been aware of an epidemic of self harm, and this report shows an increasing diversity of people using extreme ways to release their mental turmoil.' She added that self-harm is 'a potentially addictive and desperate way of dealing with the stresses of life – as one girl told us: "I need to cut myself as I need to breathe."'

In their 2006 report, *Truth Hurts*, The Camelot Foundation and Mental Health Foundation say that evidence suggests the UK has the highest rate of self-harm in Europe.

An obstacle to seeking help

Yet the difficulty with tackling self harm, as highlighted by mental health charities such as the Mental Health Foundation, is that people often hurt themselves for long periods of time without ever disclosing their self-harm. This has perhaps contributed to the lack of visibility of the issue in recent years.

The conclusions of a two-year national inquiry into self-harm, in partnership with the Camelot Foundation and the Mental Health Foundation, revealed that young people who self-harm are more likely to turn to friends their own age for help, rather than relatives, teachers or GPs. The final report, published in 2006, found that widespread misunderstandings about self-harm among professionals and relatives were preventing young people from seeking and getting support, with little information available to help parents and professionals learn to deal with self-harm appropriately and effectively.

SANE's Marjorie Wallace urges for better recognition of self-harm within the health services. Following the charity's research into self-harm, Ms Wallace said that what is 'alarming' is the numbers of those taken to A&E departments who are sent home without any follow-up help. 'We need doctors and teachers to be more alert to the potential risks, and many more therapists available, to prevent the vicious cycle of relief by painful self-harm,' she stated.

Suicidal children

The evidence for growing unhappiness among young people who strive to deal with the challenges of modern living does not stop there. Recent figures from children's charity the NSPCC reveal the number of suicidal children counselled by ChildLine has tripled in the last five years to an average of nearly 60 a week.

Of those children who gave their age, over half were aged 12 to 15 years and one in sixteen was aged 11 years or under.

On release of the figures last month, head of ChildLine, Sue Minto, commented on the reasons behind the alarming figures: 'Children feel suicidal for complex and different reasons, but often say they have a history of abuse, neglect, family problems or mental health issues. Others have been driven to the brink by bullying, their parents' divorce, the death of someone close or exam stress,' she said.

Where to turn

The Royal College of Psychiatrists advise that those who feel the need to self-harm should try to talk to someone about how they are feeling. Other ways of dealing with the emotions they experience include trying to distract yourself; writing a diary or letter to explain how you feel or trying to focus on the positive.

If you want to talk to someone, Samaritans offer non-judgmental support, 24 hours a day, seven days a week, for anyone experiencing feelings of distress or depression, which can lead to suicide. Samaritans can be contacted by phone on 08457 909090 (GB) or 1850 609090 (ROI), email at jo@samaritans.org, or face to face, visit www.samaritans.org to find your nearest branch.

⇨ The above information is reprinted with kind permission from the Samaritans. Visit www.samaritans.org for more information.

© *Samaritans*

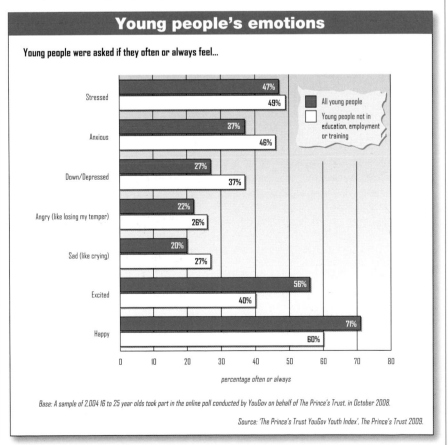

Young people's emotions

Young people were asked if they often or always feel...

- All young people
- Young people not in education, employment or training

Emotion	All young people	Young people not in education, employment or training
Stressed	47%	49%
Anxious	37%	46%
Down/Depressed	27%	37%
Angry (like losing my temper)	22%	26%
Sad (like crying)	20%	27%
Excited	56%	40%
Happy	71%	60%

percentage often or always

Base: A sample of 2,004 16 to 25 year olds took part in the online poll conducted by YouGov on behalf of The Prince's Trust, in October 2008.

Source: 'The Prince's Trust YouGov Youth Index', The Prince's Trust 2009.

Suicidal children

Children counselled by ChildLine about suicide triples

The number of suicidal children counselled by ChildLine has tripled in the last five years to an average of nearly 60 a week[1] the NSPCC reveals today (23 March 2009).

One in 14 is in immediate danger or needs urgent medical care.

Last year, nearly 3,000 children phoned ChildLine[1] because they were feeling suicidal. Some said they had attempted suicide, while others made attempts while on the phone to a counsellor.

Last year, nearly 3,000 children phoned ChildLine because they were feeling suicidal

Of those children who gave their age, over half were aged 12 to 15 years and one in sixteen was aged 11 years or under.[2]

Head of ChildLine, Sue Minto says: 'It is heartbreaking to listen to children talk of wanting to consider suicide. For a suicidal child, ChildLine can literally be a lifeline.

'Suicidal children tell us they feel utterly lonely and helpless and, apart from ChildLine, nobody seems to care whether they live or die. Our counsellors are trained to deal with suicide calls so they can assess the danger and how best to help.

'For some children, saying they want to take their own lives themselves is a cry for help, while others see it as the only way to escape their problems. While many callers will not actually attempt suicide we treat every call as extremely serious.

'Children feel suicidal for complex and different reasons, but often say they have a history of abuse, neglect, family problems or mental health issues. Others have been driven to the brink by bullying, their parents' divorce, the death of someone close or exam stress.

'Children can hide their distress so effectively that parents may have no idea their child is suicidal. We want parents to be given guidance on how to spot possible signs, how to listen to their child's worries and where to find help.

'We strongly urge any child who feels suicidal to call ChildLine. Or they could speak to a trusted adult such as their teacher or doctor.

'Every child deserves a happy childhood and the chance to grow and experience a full life. It is vital that children get the support they need.

The NSPCC also wants teachers and doctors to be trained to identify suicide distress signs before children reach crisis point.

Therapy should also be available for all children who have suffered abuse. One in five of those who called ChildLine about suicide said they had been sexually abused and nearly one in three said they had been physically abused.

Ten-year-old Sophie[3] told a Child-Line counsellor: 'I hate my life now dad's gone because I get blamed for everything and mum is in the pub every day. We never have any money because of her drinking and I've got no friends now. I just want to die.'

Another caller, thirteen-year-old Paul[3], said: 'I feel like killing myself. My mum and dad beat me and I'm getting bullied at school. I don't have anyone else to turn to except ChildLine. No one else would be able to help me. I'm scared of telling anyone.'

Four out of five calls to ChildLine about suicide were from girls and only one-fifth were from boys. But calls from boys are rising faster and are now four times higher than five years ago.

Since ChildLine joined with the NSPCC in 2006, the helpline has been expanded and answers more calls from children and young people than ever before. Even so, ChildLine is still unable to answer one in three calls.

In response, the NSPCC is urgently calling on the public to donate to its Child's Voice Appeal.[4] The charity needs to raise an extra £50 million over the next three years, in addition to £30 million already pledged by the UK Government, so that ChildLine can try to answer every call for help.

Sue Minto says: 'Children need ChildLine more than ever. We desperately need public support to help save young lives and be there for more children.'

Advice for parents

What to do if you are worried a child or young person feels suicidal:

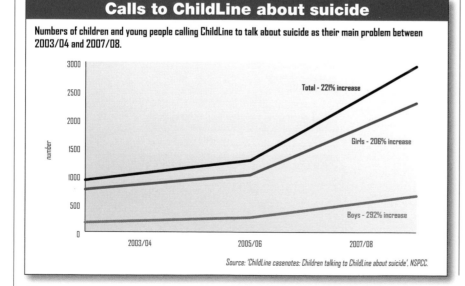

Calls to ChildLine about suicide

Numbers of children and young people calling ChildLine to talk about suicide as their main problem between 2003/04 and 2007/08.

Total - 221% increase

Girls - 206% increase

Boys - 292% increase

number

3000
2500
2000
1500
1000
500
0

2003/04   2005/06   2007/08

Source: 'ChildLine casenotes: Children talking to ChildLine about suicide'. NSPCC.

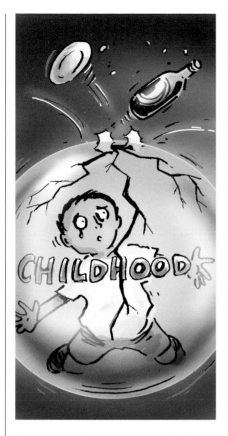

- ⇨ Acknowledge their feelings. Think about all the pressures that young people face these days from their friends, from school, from changing body shapes.
- ⇨ Be patient with them. If they respond angrily or refuse to talk to you, try and be patient with them. If they are having trouble talking to you or they get frustrated, encourage them to write down their feelings.
- ⇨ Listen to them. Listening is the single most important thing you can do in these kinds of situations. Treat what they say with respect and try not to judge them.
- ⇨ Reassure them. Tell them that they are not alone. It is common to feel upset or depressed for periods of time, but there are things they can do to make themselves feel better. Encourage them to do things that make them happy, to relax with a favourite DVD or CD, to exercise regularly to relieve stress and tension, and to get plenty of rest too.
- ⇨ Help them. Suicidal thoughts are often the result of a combination of other problems. These can include excessive drinking and taking drugs and also self-harm.
- ⇨ Tell them to call ChildLine. If they won't or can't open up to you, encourage them to call ChildLine on 0800 1111. Everything they say to a ChildLine counsellor will be confidential and ChildLine is there to listen to their problems.
- ⇨ Do not try and cope alone. You can get help and advice from your child's school nurse or doctor. There are also a number of helplines that can help you.

Notes to editors

1 In 2007/2008, a total of 2925 children and young people rang ChildLine specifically about feeling suicidal (2,282 girls and 643 boys). This has risen from 910 calls in 2003/4. The full report 'Children talking to ChildLine about suicide' will be available to download from www.nspcc.org.uk/inform from 23 March 2009.

2 72 per cent of callers gave their age.

3 Identifying details have been changed to protect the caller's identity.

4 For further information or to donate to the Child's Voice Appeal visit www.childsvoiceappeal.org.uk

23 March 2009

⇨ The above information is reprinted with kind permission from the NSPCC. Visit www.nspcc.org.uk for more information.

© NSPCC

Teens should be taught how to handle school stress

Information from the British Psychological Society

Teenagers are turning to alcohol and cigarettes to relieve school stress. This is the finding of a study presented today, 7 January 2009, at the British Psychological Society's Division of Educational and Child Psychology annual conference.

The study carried out by psychologist Dr Pamela Taylor at Salford Local Authority looked at the stressors and coping strategies of 172 15 and 16 year olds facing their GCSE examinations.

Dr Taylor said: 'Teenagers face many pressures at school – continuous achievement, examinations and having to make important decisions about their futures.'

Findings of the study indicate that the main stressors pupils experienced were the volume of coursework they were given, clashes with hand-in dates for assignments and teacher/pupil relationships. Although the majority of the pupils reported using adaptive coping strategies, such as listening to music, watching TV, sport and exercise or walking the dog, a number revealed that they engaged in forms of maladaptive coping such as drinking alcohol, smoking and taking drugs. 30 per cent drank alcohol to relieve stress, 16 per cent smoked cigarettes and six per cent used drugs.

Dr Taylor continued: 'Over a quarter of these pupils reported suffering from high levels of school-related stress. Our results illustrate how important it is to educate teenagers on the best ways to manage this stress, and highlight the dangers of using cigarettes, alcohol and drugs to cope.

'The study also shows there is a need for secondary schools to tackle pupils' school-based problems and stressors, including time management, work-life balance and teacher/pupil relationships.'

7 January 2009

⇨ The above information is reprinted with kind permission from the British Psychological Society. Visit www.bps.org.uk for more information.

© British Psychological Society

Beat exam stress

Information from the NSPCC

Plan ahead

Do

⇨ Have your own revision timetable – start planning well before exams begin. Your teacher should be able to help.

⇨ Make your books, notes and essays user-friendly. Use headings, highlighting and revision cards, and get tips on other revision techniques from teachers and friends with experience of exams. You could also consider buying revision guides.

⇨ Take notes of the important points when revising. Try to answer the questions of past exam papers – explain answers to tricky questions to someone else.

⇨ Everyone revises differently. Find out what routine suits you best – alone or with a friend or parent/carer; early morning or late at night; short, sharp bursts or longer sessions; with music or without noise.

⇨ Ask for help from your teacher/ learning mentor, parent/carer or a friend if there are things you don't understand.

Don't

⇨ Don't leave revision to the last minute.

⇨ Don't avoid revising subjects you don't like or find difficult.

⇨ Don't forget that there is life beyond revision and exams.

⇨ Don't cram ALL night before an exam.

Pamper yourself

Remember it's important to eat and sleep well. Put yourself first – this is an important time for you. Try to talk to your family about how they can make studying a little easier for you – for example, by agreeing times when you can have your own space, when they will try to be a little quieter around the house and when you'd rather not be disturbed (except perhaps for the occasional treat, such as a drink or snack).

Don't revise all the time

Make sure you give yourself time each day to relax, taking breaks to do something you enjoy – watch TV, listen to music, read a book or go out for a walk.

Prepare for the big day

⇨ Have a good breakfast if you can.

⇨ Make sure you know where the exam is being held and what time it starts. Give yourself plenty of time to get there.

⇨ Take all the equipment you need for each exam, including extra pens and pencils.

⇨ Take in a bottle of water and tissues.

⇨ Go to the loo beforehand!

If you feel really anxious, breathe slowly and deeply while waiting for the exam to start.

Pace yourself

⇨ Read the instructions before starting the exam.

⇨ Ask the teacher or exam supervisor if anything is unclear.

⇨ Read through all the questions before starting writing, and make sure you are clear how many questions you are required to answer.

⇨ If there is a choice, start by answering the question you feel you can answer best.

⇨ If you are stuck on a question, go on to the next. You can always come back to it later. If you are really stuck, try to have an intelligent guess anyway.

⇨ Leave time to read through and check your answers before the exam finishes.

⇨ Plan how much time you'll need for each question.

Perform as well as you can

⇨ Knowing that you've done your best may help you overcome feelings of letting anyone down.

⇨ Don't go through the answers afterwards with your friends if it is only going to make you more worried.

⇨ Try to put the last exam out of your mind and look ahead to the next one. You can't go back and change things. You're you, so you can only do the best you can on the day.

Phew!

Exams over? Pat yourself on the back – it's time to relax and forget about them.

If you did well – congratulations!

But remember, there's life beyond exam results. Disappointing grades are not the end of the world, even if it does feel that way at the time. You might decide to resit, and in any case, there will be lots of other

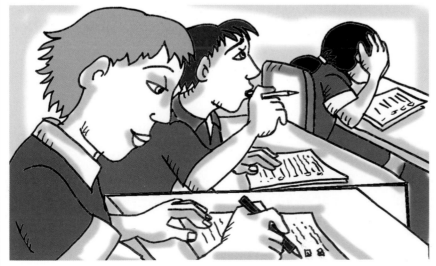

opportunities to express yourself and succeed later on in life.

Remember it's important to eat and sleep well. Put yourself first – this is an important time for you

---

Help and advice

During or after the exams, if you feel that you can't cope with the pressure or are feeling stressed, find someone to talk to. Don't bottle it up! Try to talk to your teachers, friends, or the following organisation.

ChildLine

For children and young people to call free, 24 hours a day, to talk about anything that is worrying them.

⇨ Phone: 0800 1111 (24 hours)
⇨ Textphone: 0800 400 222 (Open 9.30am to 9.30pm, Monday to Friday and 9.30am to 8pm at weekends)
⇨ Website: www.childline.org.uk

Parents and carers can help too

Ask your parents or carers to give you encouragement and support, and not to put pressure on you. Arrange with them when you can have your own quiet time and space in the house to study without being disturbed. Don't forget to talk to them if you are worried – don't bottle things up inside.

Exams are important – but they are not the only key to a successful future.

⇨ The above information is reprinted with kind permission of the NSPCC. Visit www.nspcc.org.uk for more.
© *NSPCC*

What is an eating disorder?

Information from beat

About eating disorders

Food and eating play a very important part in our lives. We all vary in the foods we like, how much we need to eat and when we like to eat. Food is essential for our health and development.

It's not unusual to experiment with different eating habits; you may have decided to become a vegetarian or tried changing your diet to improve your health. However, some eating patterns can be damaging.

Problems with food can begin when it's used to cope with those times when you are bored, anxious, angry, lonely, ashamed or sad. Food becomes a problem when it is used to help you to cope with painful situations or feelings, or to relieve stress, perhaps without you even realising it.

If this is how you deal with emotions and feelings and you are unhappy about it, then you should try to talk to someone you trust. Try not to bottle things up – this is not helpful to you or other people around you, it won't make you feel any better and the problem is unlikely to go away.

It is unlikely that an eating disorder will result from a single cause. It is much more likely to be a combination of many factors, events, feelings or pressures which lead to you feeling unable to cope. These can include: low self-esteem, family relationships,

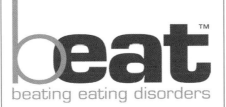

problems with friends, the death of someone special, problems at work, college or at university, lack of confidence or sexual or emotional abuse. Many people talk about simply feeling 'too fat' or 'not good enough': if you feel this way there is help available.

Often people with eating disorders say that the eating disorder is the only way they feel they can stay in control of their life, but as time goes on it isn't really you who is in control – it is the eating disorder. Some people also find they are affected by an urge to harm themselves or misuse alcohol or drugs.

You may find that in common with many other people you experience feelings of despair and shame. You may have a feeling of failure or lack of control because you cannot overcome these feelings about food on your own.

Who do eating disorders affect and when?

Anyone can develop an eating disorder, regardless of age, sex, cultural or racial background, although the people most likely to be affected tend to be young women, particularly between the ages of 15-25.

It is not unusual, however, for an eating disorder to appear in middle age. Research has shown that your genetic make-up may have a small impact upon whether or not you develop an eating disorder. In situations where there are high academic expectations, family issues or social pressures, you may focus on food and eating as a way of coping with these stresses.

'I used eating as a way of keeping control, I didn't have much confidence but felt that if I could control what I ate I could cope with everything.'

Traumatic events can sometimes trigger an eating disorder: bereavement, being bullied or abused, an upheaval in the family (such as divorce), long term illness or concerns over sexuality. Someone with a long-term illness or disability – such as diabetes, depression, blindness or deafness – may also experience eating problems.

⇨ The above information is reprinted with kind permission from beat. Visit www.b-eat.co.uk for more information.
© *beat*

⇨ Most children in England are not obese or overweight, meet the government's recommended physical activity targets, don't smoke or drink and think healthy food is enjoyable – although they're not reaching the 'five a day' target – according to the latest Health Survey for England (HSE). (page 2)

⇨ According to BMI measurements, around three in ten boys and girls aged 2-15 were either overweight or obese. (page 2)

⇨ Nearly two-thirds of premature deaths and one-third of the total disease burden in adults are associated with conditions or behaviours that began in youth, including tobacco use, a lack of physical activity, unprotected sex or exposure to violence. (page 4)

⇨ A five-year study carried out by Cancer Research UK found that physical activity declined in both teenage girls and boys, while sedentary (deskbound) activities increased. (page 7)

⇨ A new study has suggested that being overweight or seriously underweight as a teenager curbs life expectancy as much as smoking ten cigarettes a day. (page 7)

⇨ The deadliest form of skin cancer has now become the most common kind of cancer for women in their twenties – according to the latest figures from Cancer Research UK. (page 10)

⇨ In 2008 eight per cent of 11- to 15-year-old girls and five per cent of 11- to 15-year-old boys were regular smokers. (page 12)

⇨ The proportion of women who binge-drink almost doubled between 1998 and 2006 and is now at 15% (men who binge-drink increased by 1% to 23%). However, the proportion of 16- to 24-year-old men binge-drinking decreased by 9% since 2000, according to research from the Joseph Rowntree Foundation. (page 14)

⇨ The main drugs those aged 13-18 are being treated for are alcohol and/or cannabis; for 19-24 year olds it is heroin/opiates followed by cannabis and then cocaine; and for 25-30 year olds, heroin/opiates are the most common substances people in that age range are being treated for. (page 18)

⇨ Since 1995 there have been large increases in the number of people diagnosed with STIs, particularly women in their late teens and men in their early twenties. This may be because people are more aware of STIs and are visiting clinics to be tested. (page 24)

⇨ A new NHS survey shows that 16% of under-25s would not tell the person that they are sleeping with if they found out they had the STI chlamydia, while 19% are 'not sure'. (page 25)

⇨ Young people (aged 16-24 years old) are the age group most at risk of being diagnosed with a sexually transmitted infection, accounting for 65% of all chlamydia, 50% of genital warts and 50% of gonorrhoea infections diagnosed in genitourinary medicine clinics across the UK in 2007. (page 26)

⇨ 75% of sexually active youngsters are not using condoms and nearly 60% of 16 to 24 year olds questioned thought they were not at risk of contracting HIV/AIDS after having unprotected sex, according to a survey from the Staying Alive Foundation. (page 28)

⇨ Less than half of 12-18 year olds in the UK (47 per cent) think schools do enough to raise awareness of mental health issues and nearly half (43 per cent) don't believe or don't know if there is enough information available for people their age. (page 31)

⇨ One in ten 16 to 25 year olds polled by the Prince's Trust for its Youth Index study said they felt that life was meaningless, and more than a quarter (27%) said they were always or often down or depressed. Almost half of all those surveyed (47%) said they were regularly stressed. (page 32)

⇨ More than one in five 16 to 24 year olds (21%) have self-harmed, according to the results of a survey by youth mental health charity 42nd Street, youth homelessness charity Depaul UK and online communications charity YouthNet. (page 33)

⇨ The number of suicidal children counselled by ChildLine has tripled in the last five years to an average of nearly 60 a week. One in fourteen is in immediate danger or needs urgent medical care. (page 36)

⇨ A study carried out by psychologist Dr Pamela Taylor at Salford Local Authority found that 30 per cent of 15 and 16 year olds facing their GCSE examinations drank alcohol to relieve stress, 16 per cent smoked cigarettes and six per cent used drugs. (page 37)

⇨ Anyone can develop an eating disorder, regardless of age, sex, cultural or racial background, although the people most likely to be affected tend to be young women, particularly between the ages of 15-25. It is not unusual, however, for an eating disorder to appear in middle age. (page 39)

GLOSSARY

Acne
Acne consists of spots and painful bumps on the skin. It's most noticeable on the face, but can also appear on the back, shoulders and buttocks. It's caused mostly by the way skin reacts to hormonal changes, particularly during puberty.

Addiction
An addiction is a dependence on a substance which makes it very difficult to stop taking it. Addictions can be both physical and psychological.

Adolescence
The teenage years, following the onset of puberty.

Binge drinking
A recent government report describes binge drinking as 'the consumption of excessive amounts of alcohol within a limited time period', which can mean different things to different people. Another commonly used definition is 'the consumption of twice the daily benchmark given in the Government's guidelines'. This equates to six to eight alcohol units for men and four to six units for women in one sitting.

Body Mass Index (BMI)
A measurement that determines if an individual is within the healthy weight guidelines. A person's BMI is calculated by dividing their weight in kilogrammes by the square of their height in metres. For adults, a BMI between 18.5 and 25 is considered healthy. Special charts are used to calculate BMI for children, which take into account differing rates of growth and development.

Contraception
Contraception can prevent unplanned pregnancy. There are many types of contraception available to choose from, including condoms, the contraceptive pill, diaphragms, hormone injections, implants and sterilisation. Unlike non-barrier methods of contraception, using condoms can also prevent the transmission of most STIs.

Depression
Although everyone experiences feelings of sadness occasionally, for a person suffering from depression these feelings don't go away for a long period of time. Depression affects more children and young people today than in the last few decades, but it is still more common in adults. Teenagers are more likely to experience depression than young children, who rarely face depression.

Eating disorders
A group of mental health disorders that interfere with normal eating habits. Food becomes a problem when it is used to help you cope with painful situations or feelings or to relieve stress, perhaps without you even realising it. Eating disorders, including Anorexia Nervosa and Bulimia Nervosa, can cause serious health problems and even death.

Genito-urinary medicine (GUM) clinic
Genito-urinary medicine (GUM) clinics provide free checkups for sexually transmitted infections (STIs). Most STIs can be easily diagnosed and treated at GUM clinics, which are usually based in local hospitals. If you think you may have an STI, you can refer yourself to any GUM clinic for advice and treatment. The service is completely confidential and you don't have to go to your nearest clinic if you don't want to.

Obesity
A condition which occurs when an individual becomes severely overweight and their BMI exceeds 30. Obesity can cause serious health problems such as heart disease, diabetes and some types of cancer. In 2007, 17.6 per cent of 11- to 15-year-old boys and 19.0 per cent of 11- to 15-year-old girls were classed as obese.

Self-harm
Self-harm describes the different ways that people deliberately harm their bodies, to help them deal with intense emotional pain. Figures show that those aged between 11 and 25 years old are more likely to deliberately harm themselves. Those who hurt themselves deliberately often feel that physical pain is easier to deal with than the emotional pain they are experiencing.

Sexually transmitted infections (STIs)
Sexually transmitted infections (STIs) are usually passed on by sex with an infected person, though some can be passed on in other ways as well. They can be caught during oral, vaginal or anal sex. Sexually transmitted infections (STIs) are a major cause of ill health. They can also cause ectopic pregnancy (where an egg is fertilised and becomes implanted in the fallopian tube), and may also lead to infertility in both men and women. The most common sexually transmitted infection in young people is genital chlamydia.

Substance misuse
Substance misuse can refer to taking drugs or being dependent on a drug.

INDEX

accidents 4
  and alcohol 5, 15
acne 20
addiction, nicotine 13
ADHD (attention deficit hyperactivity disorder) 30
age and alcohol consumption 3, 14
age of consent 21-2
alcohol
  binge drinking 14-16
  effects of 4, 5, 15
  underage drinking 17-18
  units of 15
  and young people 3, 14, 14-18
anxiety disorders 30
attention deficit hyperactivity disorder (ADHD) 30

binge drinking 14-16
body image and exercise 7

calcium 8
calories 8
cancer, skin 10-11
ChildLine and suicidal children 35, 36-7
children
  alcohol consumption 3, 14
  health survey 2-3
  and smoking 3, 12-13
  and suicide 35, 36-7
chlamydia 25, 26
condoms 27
contraception 27
contraceptive pill 27
crime, effects of alcohol 15

depression 30, 32
  and going to university 6
diet, healthy 3, 8-9
doctors, students registering with 5
drug use 6, 18, 19
  and the law 19
  and smoking 12

eating disorders 9, 30, 39
  and going to university 6
emergency contraception 27
emotional well-being 29-39
exam stress 5, 38-9
exercise 3, 6-7

generalised anxiety disorder 30
GPs and students 5

health education and smoking 13
Health Survey for England (HSE) 2-3
healthy eating 3, 8-9

healthy lifestyles 1-20
HIV/AIDS 4
  awareness of 28

injuries, young people 4
iron intake 8

law
  and drugs 19
  and sex 21-2
  and smoking 13
  and sunbeds 11
life expectancy, effects of obesity 7

malignant melanoma 10-11
malnutrition 4
melanoma 10-11
mental health 4, 29-39
  awareness of 31-2
  risk factors 29
  treatment 30
  types of problems 30

nutrition 8-9

obesity 2, 3, 7, 9
  and health problems 7
  and life expectancy 7
  prevalence 2, 3

parents, effect on children's mental health 29-30
physical activity 3, 6-7
pill, contraceptive 27
post-traumatic stress disorder 30
pregnancy, teenage 4
protein 8

safe sex 22, 27, 28
Samaritans 35
school stress 37, 38-9
self-harm 30, 33-5
sexual health 21-8
  being ready for sex 21-2
  contraception 27
  safe sex 22, 27, 28
  sexual dysfunction 23
sexually transmitted infections (STIs) 23, 24-8
  avoiding 24, 26
skin cancer 10-11
smoking 3, 4, 12-13
  effects on appearance 11
  effects on health 12-13
  prevention 13
STIs *see* sexually transmitted infections
stress

Additional Resources

Other Issues *titles*

If you are interested in researching further some of the issues raised in *Health Issues for Young People* you may like to read the following titles in the **Issues** series:

⇨ Vol. 173 *Sexual Health* (ISBN 978 1 86168 487 5)

⇨ Vol. 170 *Body Image and Self-Esteem* (ISBN 978 1 86168 484 4)

⇨ Vol. 164 *The AIDS Crisis* (ISBN 978 1 86168 468 4)

⇨ Vol. 163 *Drugs in the UK* (ISBN 978 1 86168 456 1)

⇨ Vol. 162 *Staying Fit* (ISBN 978 1 86168 455 4)

⇨ Vol. 145 *Smoking Trends* (ISBN 978 1 86168 411 0)

⇨ Vol. 143 *Problem Drinking* (ISBN 978 1 86168 409 7)

⇨ Vol. 141 *Mental Health* (ISBN 978 1 86168 407 3)

⇨ Vol. 140 *Vegetarian and Vegan Diets* (ISBN 978 1 86168 406 6)

⇨ Vol. 136 *Self-Harm* (ISBN 978 1 86168 388 5)

⇨ Vol. 133 *Teen Pregnancy and Lone Parents* (ISBN 978 1 86168 379 3)

⇨ Vol. 128 *The Cannabis Issue* (ISBN 978 1 86168 374 8)

⇨ Vol. 127 *Eating Disorders* (ISBN 978 1 86168 366 3)

⇨ Vol. 125 *Understanding Depression* (ISBN 978 1 86168 364 9)

⇨ Vol. 100 *Stress and Anxiety* (ISBN 978 1 86168 314 4)

⇨ Vol. 88 *Food and Nutrition* (ISBN 978 1 86168 289 5)

For more information about these titles, visit our website at www.independence.co.uk/publicationslist

Useful organisations

You may find the websites of the following organisations useful for further research:

⇨ **ASH:** www.ash.org.uk

⇨ **AVERT:** www.avert.org

⇨ **beat:** www.b-eat.co.uk

⇨ **British Heart Foundation:** www.bhf.org.uk

⇨ **The British Psychological Society:** www.bps.org.uk

⇨ **Brook:** www.brook.org.uk

⇨ **Cancer Research UK:** www.cancerresearchuk.org

⇨ **ChildLine:** www.childline.org.uk

⇨ **Food Standards Agency:** www.food.gov.uk

⇨ **Health Protection Agency:** www.hpa.org.uk

⇨ **Institute of Child Health:** www.ich.ucl.ac.uk

⇨ **Mental Health Foundation:** www.mentalhealth.org.uk

⇨ **NHS Choices:** www.nhs.uk

⇨ **NSPCC:** www.nspcc.org.uk

⇨ **Samaritans:** www.samaritans.org

⇨ **TheSite:** www.thesite.org

⇨ **Terrence Higgins Trust:** www.tht.org.uk

⇨ **World Health Organization:** www.who.int

⇨ **YouthNet:** www.youthnet.org

ACKNOWLEDGEMENTS

The publisher is grateful for permission to reproduce the following material.

While every care has been taken to trace and acknowledge copyright, the publisher tenders its apology for any accidental infringement or where copyright has proved untraceable. The publisher would be pleased to come to a suitable arrangement in any such case with the rightful owner.

Chapter One: Healthy Lifestyles

Health questionnaire, © Crown copyright is reproduced with the permission of Her Majesty's Stationery Office, How healthy are our children?, © NatCen, Adolescent health, © WHO, 'Is drinking too much really that big a deal?', © Guardian News & Media Ltd 2008, What's the best exercise for teenagers?, © Crown copyright is reproduced with the permission of Her Majesty's Stationery Office, Being obese is as bad as a packet of cigarettes, © British Heart Foundation 2009, Good nutrition during the teenage years, © Tesco, Skin cancer now threatens women in their twenties, © Cancer Research UK, Young smokers fear future impact on their appearance, © British Psychological Society, Young people and smoking, © ASH, Alcohol in Britain, © Joseph Rowntree Foundation, Binge drinking, © TheSite, Britain's 'chronic' teenage binge-drinking problem, © Telegraph Media Group Limited (2009), London 2009, Underage drinking debate, © Headliners, More young people seek help for problems with drugs, © NTA, Drug problems, © Crown copyright is reproduced with the permission of Her Majesty's Stationery Office, Acne, © Crown copyright is reproduced with the permission of Her Majesty's Stationery Office.

Chapter Two: Sexual Health

Am I ready for sex?, © AVERT, Healthy sex life, © Terrence Higgins Trust, Sexually transmitted infections, © Brook, Sex secrets putting young people's health at risk, © Westminster PCT, STIs and young people, © HPA, Contraception – the facts, © r u thinking?, Concern over young people's risky sex, © Guardian News & Media Ltd 2009.

Chapter Three: Mental Health

Children and young people, © Mental Health Foundation, Young people's mental health ignorance, © Institute of Child Health, Depression among the young at alarming level, © Guardian News & Media Ltd 2009, One in five young people have self-harmed, © YouthNet, The epidemic of self-harm, © Samaritans, Suicidal children, © NSPCC, Teens should be taught how to handle school stress, © British Psychological Society, Beat exam stress, © NSPCC, What is an eating disorder?, © beat.

Photographs

Stock Xchng: pages 11, 30 (Sanja Gjenero); 15 (mark, Watje11, Andrzej Gdula, Nathan Bauer, Laura Nubuck); 26 (Patti Adair).
Wikimedia Commons: page 18 (Chmee2).

Illustrations

Pages 1, 13, 20, 33: Don Hatcher; pages 5, 17, 28: Angelo Madrid; pages 2, 16, 24, 37: Simon Kneebone; pages 10, 38: Bev Aisbett.

Editorial and layout by Claire Owen, on behalf of Independence Educational Publishers.

And with thanks to the team: Mary Chapman, Sandra Dennis, Claire Owen and Jan Sunderland.

Lisa Firth
Cambridge
September, 2009